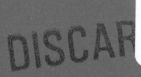

EVERYTHING EYES

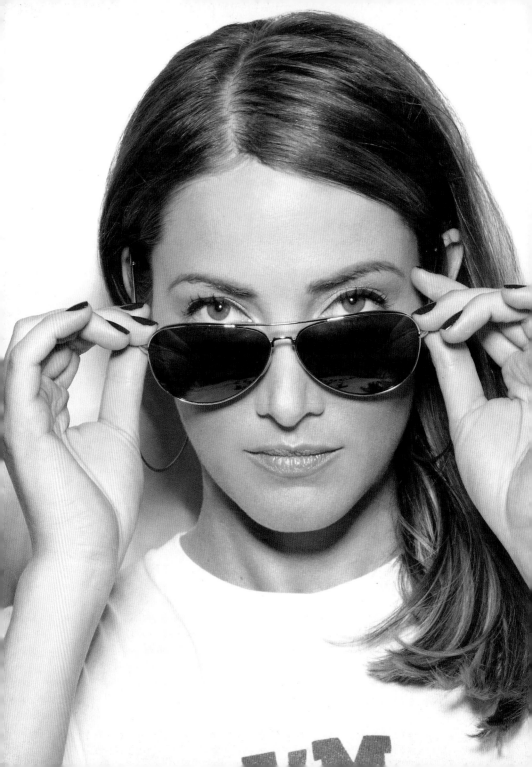

EVERYTHING EYES

PROFESSIONAL TECHNIQUES
ESSENTIAL TOOLS
GORGEOUS MAKEUP LOOKS

BOBBI BROWN

WITH SARA BLISS

CHRONICLE BOOKS

SAN FRANCISCO

Library of Congress Cataloging-in-Publication Data available.

ISBN: 978-1-4521-1961-8

Manufactured in China

Designed by Pamela Geismar

10 9 8 7 6 5 4 3 2

Chronicle Books LLC
680 Second Street
San Francisco, California 94107
www.chroniclebooks.com

CONTENTS

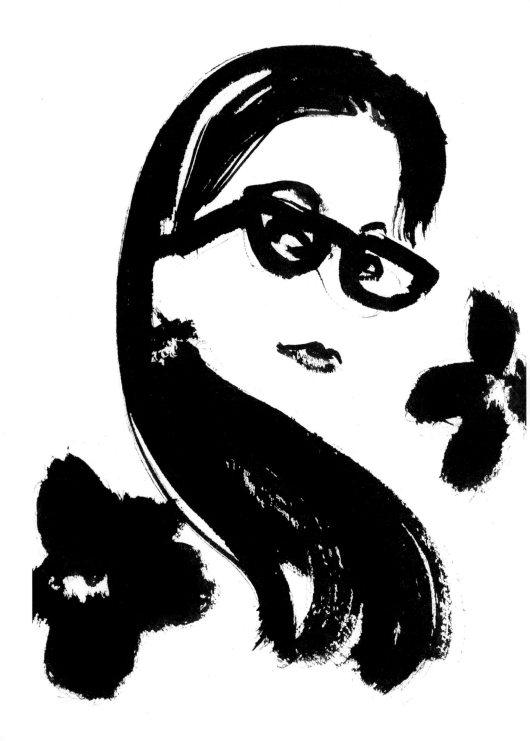

INTRODUCTION

I wrote this book to teach you how simple it is to make up your eyes. Once you master the basic techniques, the rest is actually pretty easy. With *Everything Eyes*, you'll be able to achieve beautiful eyes that pop in a few steps. First, I'll show you how to work with the right tools and products. Then, we'll move on to ten of my go-to eye-makeup looks, from sparkly to smokey to retro glam. If, like me, you wear glasses, you will learn how to choose the perfect pair (or two) and how to make your eyes stand out from under your lenses.

All of the models in this book are real girls whose transformations are both stunning and achievable. Now you can rock amazing eyes, too.

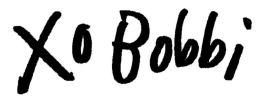

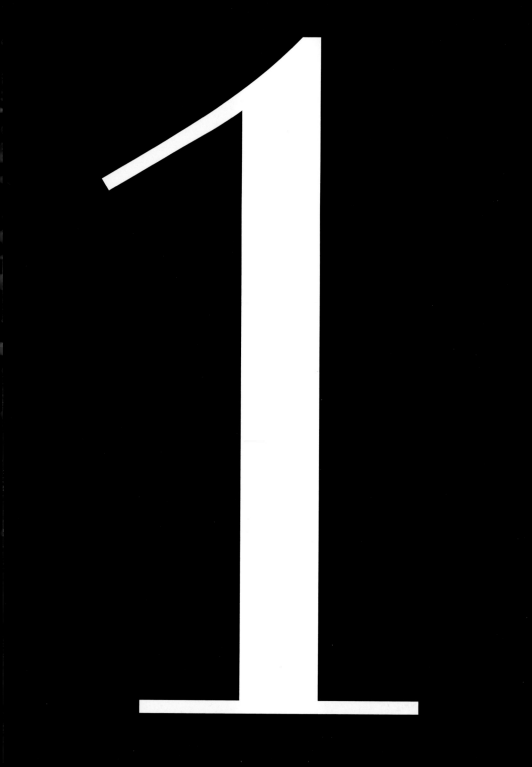

the basics

With the right tools and simple makeup techniques, anyone can be their own makeup artist and create stand-out eyes.

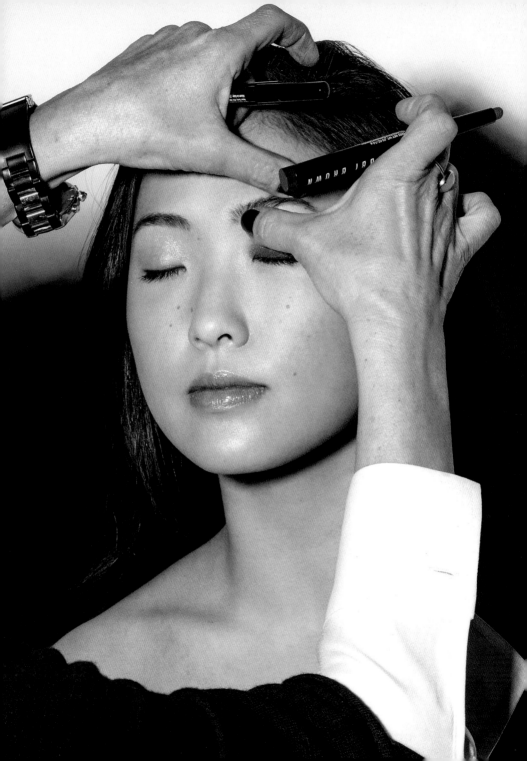

brushes and tools

The right tools make all the difference. This is especially true when applying eye makeup. Whether it's getting concealer to blend in, creating a smokey eye, or drawing the perfect line, using the correct brush or tool is key.

There are five essential brushes that I recommend: a concealer brush, a fuller eye sweep brush, a rounded eye shadow brush with natural bristles, a flat eyeliner brush, and a brow brush. These five will help you create a beautiful, classic eye. If you want to try more advanced techniques, add a few more brushes to your beauty arsenal. This glossary will help you decide exactly what you need to create the look you want. Good brushes make creating stunning eyes that much easier.

THE FIVE ESSENTIAL BRUSHES

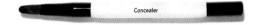

CONCEALER BRUSH

This is a tapered flat brush that lets you place the right amount of undereye concealer only where you need it. The fine tip is designed to reach tricky spots like the inner corners of eyes. While concealer brushes should be firm, it is important that the bristles be soft, not scratchy, because of how delicate the skin around your eyes is.

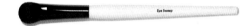

EYE SWEEP BRUSH

This full, rounded brush is the perfect multitasker. Use it to apply shadow over the entire lid, the lower lid, or even the crease.

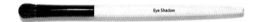

ROUNDED EYE SHADOW BRUSH

The ideal brush for sweeping shadow across the lower lid is a medium brush with a rounded edge and soft, natural bristles. Beveled edges beautifully layer and blend color.

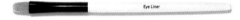

EYELINER BRUSH (FLAT)

This brush can be used wet or dry to create the perfect line whether you prefer your liner thin or thick.

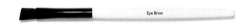

BROW BRUSH

A brush with angled bristles helps deposit just the right amount of powder shadow to define and enhance brows.

À LA CARTE BRUSHES

EYE SMUDGE BRUSH

The best tool for creating a smokey eye, this small brush is amazing for layering color on the lower lid and in the crease. It is also small enough to smudge liner.

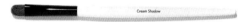

EYE BLENDER BRUSH

An eye blender brush with long, soft bristles gently blends shadows together for a beautiful finish. Because of its light touch, you can also use it for setting concealer with face powder.

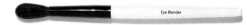

CREAM SHADOW BRUSH

Cream shadows require special synthetic bristles. This small brush is designed to work with all of my long-wear shadows, distributing the perfect amount.

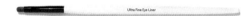

EYELINER BRUSH (ULTRA FINE)

To create an expert line with liquid or gel eyeliner, look for a slim, tapered brush. Synthetic bristles help liquid liner glide smoothly on the eyelid.

✻ a few thoughts on bristles

With natural and synthetic bristles, one isn't better than the other. It all depends on what type of makeup you are using. Here's what you need to know about both kinds.

NATURAL

Cruelty-free natural bristles made from pony or goat are the ideal material for working with powder shadows or liners. They deposit the right amount of powder and make it easy to blend colors and soften lines.

SYNTHETIC

Cream-based products such as gel liner, cream shadows, concealer, and corrector require stiff, precise bristles made from synthetic fibers. Unlike natural bristles, which will be ruined by creamy products, these versions are designed to handle and apply liquid-based makeup.

✻ maintaining your brushes

Your brushes can last for years if you clean them every few weeks. Here's how.

- Start by placing a couple of drops of brush cleanser, mild soap, or baby shampoo in your palm.
- Add a tiny amount of water to the brush and place the bristles in the soap in your palm, working up a lather on the brush.
- Very gently rinse with warm water.
- Dry off with a paper towel or a dry cloth and reshape the brush.
- Let the brush dry hanging off the edge of a counter.

OTHER USEFUL TOOLS

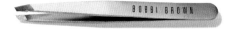

TWEEZERS

There is nothing more frustrating than trying to wield a pair of tweezers that just don't work. Invest in a good pair that is wide enough for an easy grip and slanted to a fine point, making it easy to pluck even the finest hairs.

BROW GROOMING BRUSH

Stiff, flat brushes help quickly groom brows into place for a neat, polished look. Brushing brows is a step people often ignore, but it really makes a difference in your look.

EYELASH CURLER

A foolproof way to instantly open your eyes, an eyelash curler extends and curls lashes before you put on mascara. Look for versions that are easy to grip, have cushioned pads, and shape the lashes into a natural-looking curl. Always curl lashes before applying mascara to avoid breaking them.

YOUR FINGERS

One of the best eye makeup tools you have is your fingers. The warmth of your fingers helps makeup blend more easily into your skin, making corrector and concealer look more natural. And because the skin picks up color more intensely than a brush, your fingers can provide a denser, stronger application of eye shadow color. When you have finished applying your eye makeup with brushes, rely on your hands for touch-ups such as blending shadow, correcting liner, and removing stray powder.

healthy eyes

Achieving gorgeous eyes is about more than just makeup. Your sleep habits, nutrition, and the ingredients in your products all play a part in how great your eyes look.

Lifestyle also counts. Too much sodium and alcohol, stress, smoking, or lack of sleep will all show up in the form of dark circles, bags, and even wrinkles. Avoid those triggers and you will notice a big difference in your eyes. Drinking more water, eating lots of fruits and vegetables, avoiding processed salty foods, going to bed earlier, and exercising regularly will do more to give you beautiful, bright eyes than any cream or makeup can.

✳ the doctor says

It's a fact of life that everyone's eyesight starts to decline at age forty. The good news is that you can target a variety of eye issues with better nutrition and good eye habits. I asked my ophthalmologists, Dr. Tanya Carter and Dr. Frank Barnes, Jr., to share their tips for taking care of your eyes.

GO EASY

Always read with good lighting and from a healthy working distance. Don't hold reading material or electronic devices closer than elbow length from your eyes. Be sure to rest eyes every thirty minutes by looking up from your task and focusing your eyes on a distant target.

KEEP YOUR EYES CLEAR

Manage eye redness by treating underlying causes like lack of sleep or dryness, rather than reaching for over-the-counter eyedrops. The drops can actually make your eyes more red and irritated over time.

FOCUS ON NUTRITION

Boosting your nutrients can help manage conditions such as macular degeneration, glaucoma, diabetic retinopathy, and lipid tear deficiency dry eye. Antioxidant-rich foods that include vitamins A, C, and E and zinc help maintain retinal cells. Kale, spinach, broccoli, and dark green lettuces contain carotenoids such as lutein and zeaxanthin that help protect the retina against UV damage and are associated with improved visual acuity and contrast sensitivity. Omega-3 essential fatty acids found in fish, or taken in pill form, help prevent dry eye and promote healthy retinal function.

WHAT TO LOOK FOR IN EYE CREAM

Whether you want to tackle dark circles, puffiness, crow's-feet, or wrinkles, there are products to help. The best creams and serums boast special ingredients that target your trouble spots. Here are a few key ingredients to look for.

ALOE VERA

The best sunburn treatment around is also known for soothing the driest, most inflamed skin. When you want to hydrate, calm, and nourish skin, look for products that include aloe.

ANTIOXIDANTS

Green tea extract; vitamins A, C, and E; and grape seed extract are proven to neutralize free radicals (highly charged oxygen molecules caused by sun, smoking, and stress that can cause inflammation, loss of collagen, wrinkles, and dark spots). Antioxidants counteract free radical damage and boost cell repair, fade discoloration and blotches, and stimulate collagen production.

CAFFEINE

Drink too much caffeine and you can dehydrate your skin. But as an ingredient in eye creams, caffeine is a total beauty enhancer. Caffeine has been shown to reduce puffiness, tighten skin, and minimize dark circles.

GREEN TEA EXTRACT

Studies have shown that green tea extract is one of the most effective antioxidants at neutralizing free radicals and is an especially potent anti-aging ingredient.

HYALURONIC ACID

This is the ingredient for thirsty eyes. Hyaluronic acid works to plump up skin and boost skin cells with extra moisture.

PEPTIDES

Peptides increase collagen and elastin production to help keep wrinkles at bay. They are also extremely gentle, making them a good choice if you have sensitive skin.

VITAMIN C

Because vitamin C is proven to increase the production of collagen and elastin, it is a powerful tool against wrinkles. Look for formulas that use ascorbic acid and are paired with vitamin E to boost its effectiveness.

VITAMIN E

A powerful antioxidant that repairs, protects, and moisturizes, vitamin E also has incredibly soothing and calming properties.

a word about retinol

Retinol, a potent vitamin A derivative, is considered one of the most effective ways to treat fine lines, wrinkles, and sunspots. Retinol stimulates cell turnover and increases collagen production. However, it can only be used at night because it interacts poorly with sunlight. If you have very sensitive skin you should avoid retinol completely, as it can trigger redness and rashes.

NATURAL EYE TREATMENTS

Sometimes the best eye treatments are the simplest. When it comes to bloating and puffiness in your face, nothing beats avoiding salty meals and drinking a few cups of lemon- or cranberry-infused water. You can also find some of nature's best eye beauty boosters just by opening up your fridge or reaching into the pantry. Following are a few.

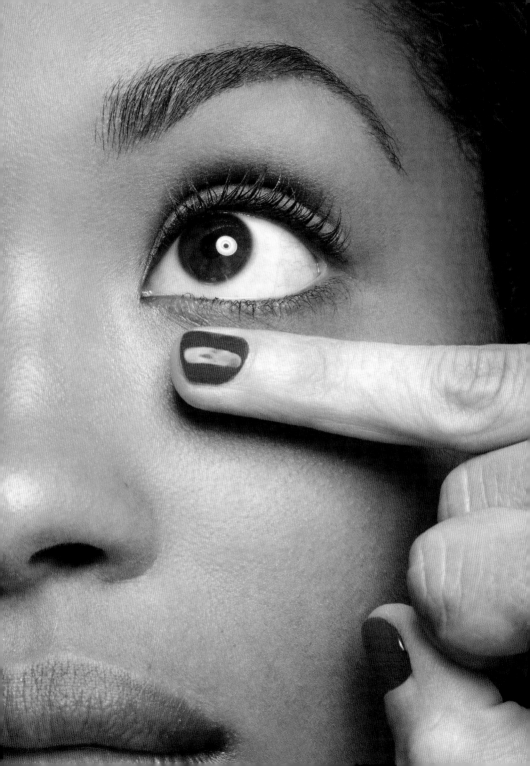

COLD TEA BAGS

Rough night? Tea bags will help. Steep them in hot water for five minutes, wring them out, and cool in the fridge. Lie back with your head elevated and the cold tea bags placed on your eyes. The caffeine in green or black tea will help reduce swelling, while chamomile calms redness and irritation.

CUCUMBERS

Yes, it's true: Sliced cold cucumbers placed on eyes are amazing at de-puffing and reducing irritation thanks to their cool temperature and astringent properties.

JOJOBA OIL

Applied with a cotton ball, jojoba oil is a very effective and hydrating natural makeup remover. It easily removes shadow and liner, and makes a great moisturizer in a pinch.

SLEEPING WITH YOUR HEAD ELEVATED

A pillow that keeps the head and neck supported and elevated helps promote lymphatic drainage, making sure that fluid doesn't settle in the skin around your eyes. While sleeping flat on your back might be fine for your back, it's not good for puffiness.

TAKE IT OFF

Because the eye area is so delicate, you should only take off your makeup with a remover specifically designed for eyes. I recommend gentle formulas that include soothing ingredients such as aloe vera and rosewater extract. If you wear waterproof or long-wear eye makeup, you will need a product formulated to remove long-lasting makeup.

The best way to apply eye makeup remover is with a cotton ball or pad. A cotton swab can finish off any extra traces.

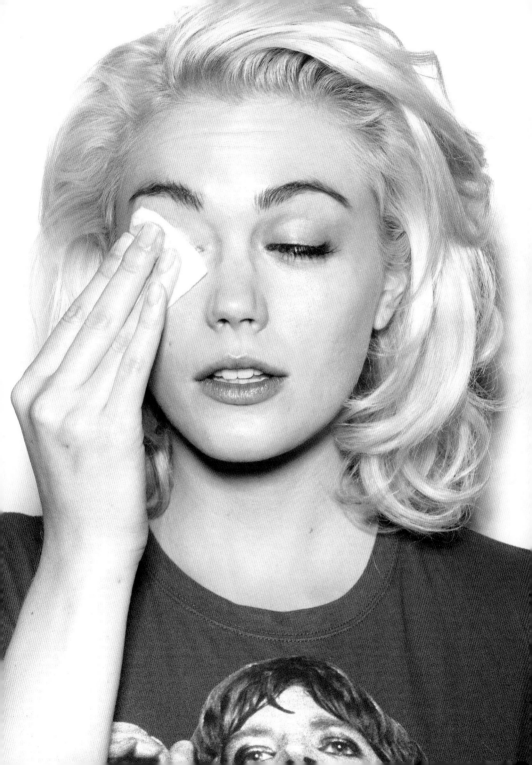

✱ the doctor says

There are so many amazing products out there for eyes. However, it can be hard to navigate all your options. I asked dermatologist Dr. Rosemarie Ingleton for advice on alleviating the three most common beauty complaints.

DARK CIRCLES
Eye creams with vitamin K work to combat undereye darkness.

PUFFINESS
Products with caffeine, green tea extract, chamomile, and Matrixyl (an antiaging ingredient) are best.

WRINKLES
Look for products that contain retinol, alpha hydroxy acids, Matrixyl, hyaluronic acid, neuropeptides, and growth factors.

✱ ask a product developer

HOW LONG DO I KEEP EYE MAKEUP?
We asked Gabrielle Nevin, VP of Global Product Development at Bobbi Brown Cosmetics, how long you should keep your favorite products before updating them. Here's what she shared.

- Face powder and powder eye shadow: Two years
- Eyeliner: Two years
- Mascara: Six months
- Corrector and concealer: Two years
- Eye creams: Six months
- Brushes: More than 10 years with proper care (see page 15)

In the event of an eye infection, you may need to toss any makeup that came into contact with the infection. It's best to consult your doctor.

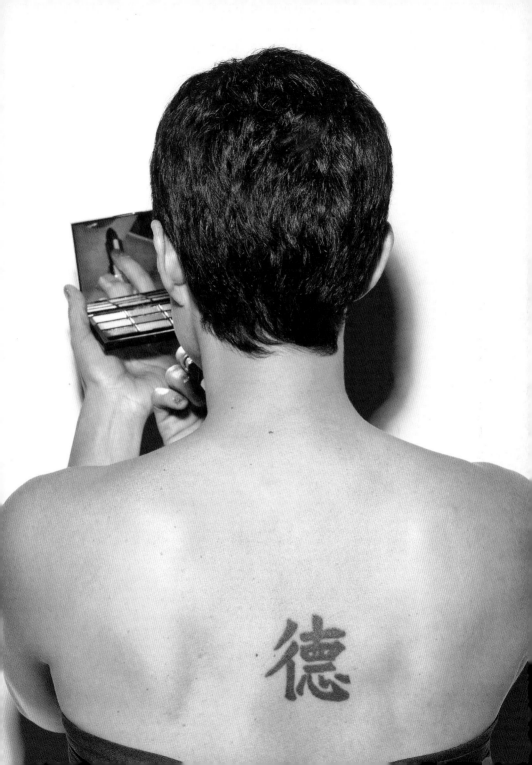

basic eye techniques

From how to banish undereye circles with concealer and corrector to making your eyes pop with liner, here are my foolproof tips for achieving gorgeous eyes.

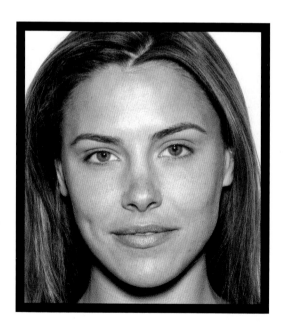

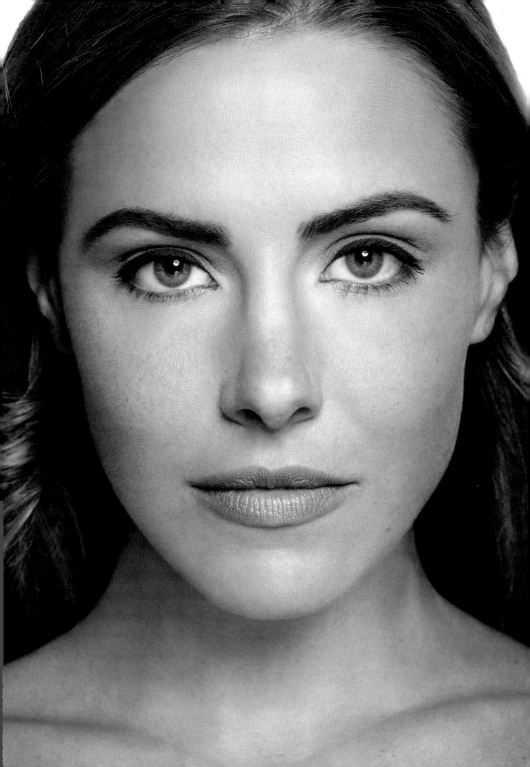

corrector

I frequently get asked what is the one type of makeup that I absolutely can't live without. My answer is always corrector and concealer. They are the products that can most dramatically improve the way you look. When you apply corrector and concealer, you appear less tired, more refreshed, and instantly brighter. That's why I call them the secret of the universe. The combination of both products make them the rock stars of any woman's makeup bag.

If you have chronic dark circles, or maybe just had a late night, layer corrector underneath concealer. Corrector is a pink- or peach-based undereye makeup designed to neutralize, brighten, and counteract discoloration around the eye.

CHOOSING YOUR SHADE OF CORRECTOR

Pink- or bisque-toned correctors work for women with pale to medium skin. Women with warmer skin tones should look for peach corrector. Darker peach or dark bisque corrector works on darker skin tones. If your corrector appears too white after application, it's not the right shade; go darker. If it's too yellow or doesn't instantly brighten, go lighter.

APPLYING CORRECTOR

Start by applying a small amount of quick-absorbing eye cream. Then, apply corrector with a brush to the inner corner of the eye area, placing it only where you see darkness. Then, gently blend with your fingers. Next, clean your brush with a tissue before applying concealer— corrector and concealer don't work if they are mixed together, they work when layered.

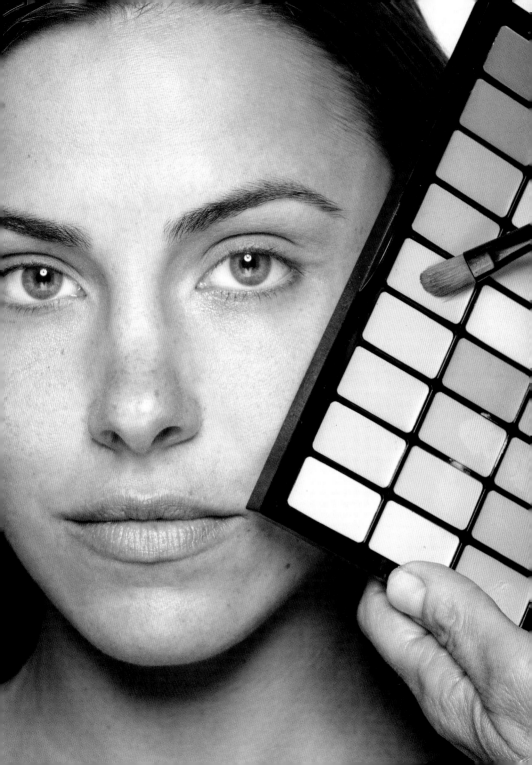

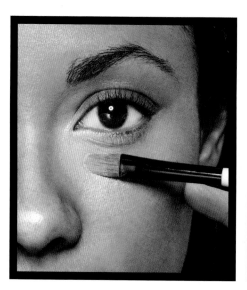
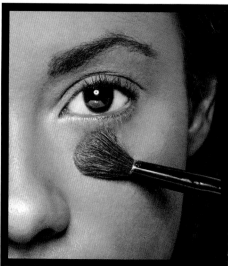

CORRECTOR & CONCEALER TIPS

- Always use a small amount of hydrating eye cream before applying corrector and concealer. Make sure the cream absorbs into your skin and is not too greasy, otherwise your makeup will slide right off.

- Your skin color often varies from winter to summer. If you change to a slightly darker foundation in the summer, you may need a slightly darker concealer as well.

- Layer and pat the concealer with your fingers to help blend it into the skin. Never tug or pull at the delicate skin around the eyes—dab and softly blend.

- Pale yellow or white sheer powder on top of concealer will set it in place.

concealer

Yellow-based concealers work magic when applied over corrector with a clean brush. They lighten the dark areas, cover up redness, and instantly make you look rested. They brighten your eye area, giving an immediate lift.

CHOOSING YOUR SHADE OF CONCEALER

To pick the right shade of concealer, look for a yellow-based creamy formula that is one shade lighter than your natural skin tone. Women of all skin tones benefit from a yellow-based formula. The yellow blends well into the skin, making you look awake without looking like you're wearing a lot of makeup.

APPLYING CONCEALER

With a clean brush, apply concealer on top of corrector, making sure to go close to the eyelashes and in the inner corner and socket of the eyes. Blend with your fingers until it appears smooth.

FINISH WITH POWDER

Set concealer with powder to keep it from creasing and make it last even longer. Simply apply a light dusting of yellow-toned powder over concealer with an eye sweep brush. If you are very pale, try translucent powder. Go with peach-based powder if you have a darker skin type.

TROUBLESHOOTING

If, after applying corrector and concealer, it looks dry under your eyes, you didn't start out with enough eye cream. If anything smears, you likely applied too much cream and should add more powder to finish.

brows

Beautifully arched eyebrows really frame the eye and add both polish and definition. They also provide an instant eye lift.

SHAPING BROWS

To get the right brow shape for your face, see a professional first. Even if you have already over-tweezed or have created uneven brows, an expert will be able to guide you to achieving the right shape. Once that shape is established you can keep it up on your own by tweezing hairs as they grow back in. When you are grooming your own brows, your best tools are a pair of professional-quality tweezers and a shadow pencil.

DEFINING BROWS

Defining your brows really completes your look. It is a step that is often overlooked, but once you start doing it you will wonder why you didn't.

Begin by taking a stiff angled brow brush and eye shadow in the same tone as your hair and/or brow color. Apply from the inner corner of your brows and brush straight up. For the rest of the brow, brush up and over and work your way from the inner corner through the arch and on to the end with light strokes, filling in any gaps with powder.

If your brows are messy and unruly, apply a clear brow shaper after color application. This mascara-like wand with liquid color both tames and defines brows. For a subtle look, you can simply brush up your brows with a product like my Natural Brow Shaper.

BROW COLOR TIPS

- Your brow color should match your hair color, but if you have black hair go with a slightly softer shade such as a deep brown-black. If you are blonde, keep brows lighter but in the same tone as your hair.

- If you have bare spots that aren't fixed with powder, fill them in with a brow pencil in the same tone as your hair or brows.

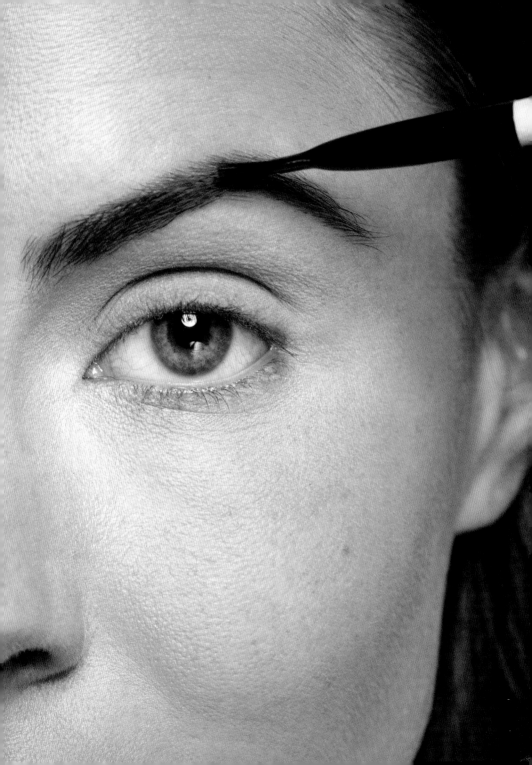

eye shadow

Every woman should know how to do an easy, classic eye using two shadows that work with her skin tone. Pair this eye shadow look with liner and mascara and you will always look pretty and amazing.

CHOOSING EYE SHADOW COLORS

For a basic eye, start with a light shadow as your base. It should lighten your lid and be almost, but not quite, invisible. You want to go with a color that enhances your natural skin tone without looking too ashy, pink, or gray. Women with fair skin should look for white or bone shades, while women with darker complexions should choose banana- or peachy-toned shadows. In a basic eye, the medium shadow should be one shade darker than your skin tone. Beige, soft brown, or gray shadows are nice choices for fair skin, while camel or rich browns are right for women with darker skin.

APPLYING EYE SHADOW

Achieving a beautiful classic eye with shadow can be done in two steps. Simply take an eye shadow brush and apply a light powder base color all over the lid, from the lash line to the brow bone.

Next, apply your medium shade with a shadow brush from the lash line to the crease, all across the lower lid. For additional depth, you can add a third, slightly darker color into the crease, blending just above and below the crease.

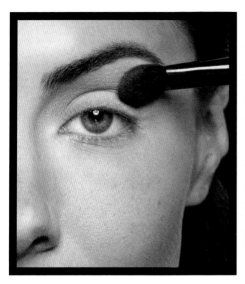
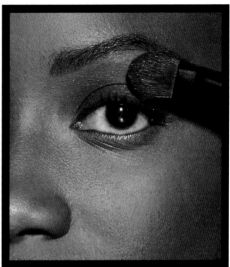

EYE SHADOW TIPS

- If you have redness around your eyes, stay away from shadows with red or purple undertones as these colors will exacerbate the redness.

- For a foolproof eye, layer shadows from light to dark. Start with the palest shadow as the base, then layer a medium shade, and apply the darkest shade last.

- Powder shadows are great for beginners. They blend more easily than cream shadows and are easy to correct if you make a mistake. Cream shadows allow for a denser application.

- There are no rules for how many shadow colors you need to create a beautiful eye. Sometimes one amazing color is all you need.

eyeliner

From pencil to powder to gels, there are many formulas of eyeliner. Each creates a different effect. Gel liner can be dramatic and long-wearing, while powder can be softer and more subtle. If you make a mistake, just dip a cotton swab in eye makeup remover, take off the liner, and begin again. During the day, you should be able to correct any smudges with a cotton swab or tissue. Makeup artist Cassandra Garcia is a wiz with liner. I asked her to share her techniques for applying every kind of liner.

POWDER LINER

Powder shadow offers one of the easiest, most foolproof ways to line your eyes. Applied dry, the line will be softer and more diffused. Applied damp, the liner will be stronger and longer-lasting.

The thickness of the line depends on the type of brush you use and how bold you want your look. The thicker the liner, the bolder the look. A flat eyeliner brush is great for powder liner; you can easily build up your line from very thin to thick.

To apply liner, start from the outer corner working your way in toward the inner corner. Make sure you go as close to the lash line as possible without any gap. Draw the line all the way to the inner corner so the line looks smooth.

APPLICATION TIPS

- To make sure your liner pops, always apply liner after eye shadow.

- The thickest part of the line should always be on the outside corner of the eye, while the thinnest is at the inner corner. This trick visually lifts the eye and highlights your eye shape.

- Make sure you can see the top line when your eye is open. If not, the line is too thin. This is especially important on deep-set and Asian eyes.

- If you also line the bottom lash line, remember that it should be a much softer line than on your upper lid.

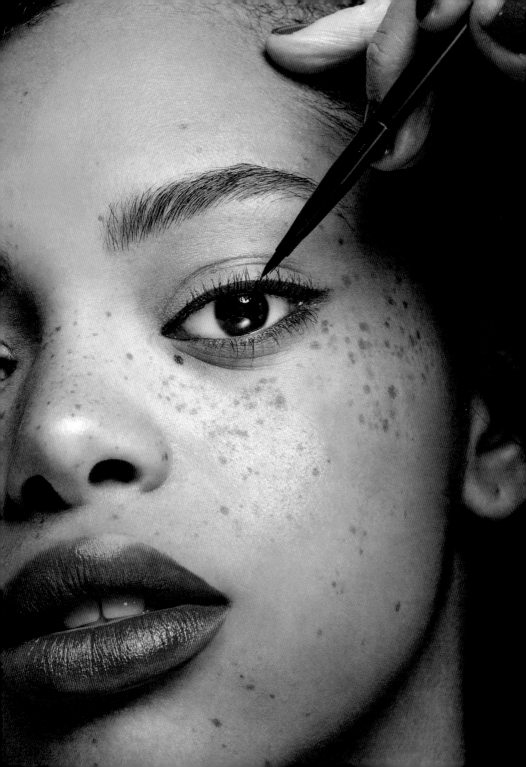

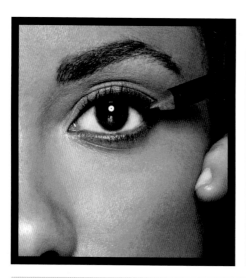
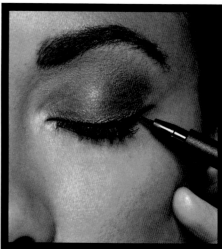

EYELINER TIPS

- If you have a lot of undereye darkness, skip lining the lower lash line as it will only draw attention to the problem. Instead, just use waterproof mascara on the lower lashes.

- The top and bottom lines should connect at the outer corner of your eye. This best defines your eye's natural shape.

- Always line all the way across from the outer corner to the inner corner. Never line only halfway.

- To soften the line, just use your finger or a cotton swab to smudge slightly.

- Powder liner can soften a too-harsh gel liner and make it look diffused.

- Gel or ink pen liner on top of a powder liner helps create a sexy, smokey eye with a clean sharp edge.

- Here's a great trick if you like the look of the pencil but find it hard to apply: Take a liner brush and use it to pick up color from your pencil, then apply with the brush. This will create a more intense line than just dry powder, but will be easier to apply than pencil.

PENCIL LINER

The newest pencil liners are long-wear versions designed to stay on all day—no streaking, no smearing. You will be able to create a thin precise line or, if you go with a kajal liner, a slightly smudged, sexy look.

To apply liner, draw the pencil across the lash line, starting from the outer corner in. Line your way across the lash line until your line is smooth and even. Make sure there are no gaps between the liner and lash line. If you want a softer effect, use your finger or a brush to smudge.

For added definition, you can also line the lower lash line using the same technique going from outer to inner corner. It is important that you connect the upper and lower lines at the outer corner of your eye.

GEL LINER

Gel liner provides a clean, crisp line. It also offers the densest color you can get. Smudge-proof and water-resistant, gel liner lasts all day so it's perfect for day-to-night. Double lining with a gel first, then smudging with a powder liner will create a look that is even more dramatic.

To use, you will need a synthetic bristle brush designed for working with gel formulas. For the best control, choose a small, slim, tapered brush.

Dip the tip of the brush into the pot to capture the gel. Begin by applying the liner very close to the lash line from the outer corner in. If there's a gap between the eyeliner and your lash line, fill it in with extra liner.

Gel can also be used for lining just under the top lid (this is called underlining) for added drama. Gel can be too harsh for the lower lash line; try pencil instead.

INK LINER

Ink eyeliner combines the intensity of a gel liner with an easy-to-use applicator that is almost like a pen. It's ideal if you want to create winged liner (see page 64) or a more defined line.

Using the tip, apply the liner in long, smooth strokes from the outer corner in.

lashes

For a quick and easy way to define and open up your eyes, mascara is an everyday essential. Different formulas deliver different benefits, including lengthening, thickening, and enhancing lashes. Long-wear or waterproof versions can stay on for up to twelve hours.

Choose a mascara based on your needs. Skimpy lashes benefit from a lengthening formula. Sparse lashes need a thickening option. Volumizing versions enhance lashes. You can layer two different mascara formulas for maximum effect. The goal is to work with the lashes you have to achieve the lashes you want.

For color, I almost always choose the blackest of black mascara. If you want a more subtle look, try dark brown.

CURLING

A lash curler is a great tool to open up the eyes. It isn't an essential step, but it does create a more dramatic eye. If you have lashes that stick straight out or point downward it will really help.

Always curl lashes before you apply mascara, otherwise you may break your lashes. Crimp at the base of the lashes, then hold the curler for five to ten seconds as you lift up and let go. Just once is enough.

For a quick pick-me-up you can just use your fingers, holding the lashes in a curl with your fingertips for a few seconds.

APPLYING MASCARA

Hold the wand horizontally and start at the base of the lashes. Roll the wand as you go up to the tip of your lashes to help separate and avoid clumps. Repeat once or twice (no need to let lashes dry between coats). Before lashes dry, gently press them up with your fingers to curl them and open your eyes up even more.

For slightly more definition, apply mascara to the lower lashes but use a much lighter touch and only one coat.

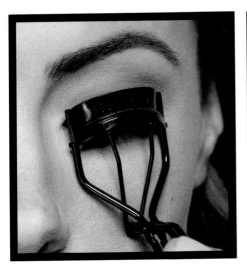

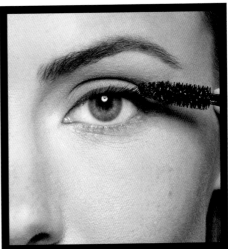

MASCARA TIPS

- Always curl lashes before applying mascara.

- To avoid smearing mascara, make sure there isn't too much moisture on your lid or undereye area. If you are using a cream shadow or a gel or ink liner, make sure that the makeup has dried before you coat your lashes. Always set your concealer with powder so the area under the eye is dry.

- The best way to take off mascara is with a tissue or cotton pad and eye makeup remover. Blot rather than rub it off.

- Always put the top wand back and tighten the cap to keep mascara fresh.

- Replace mascara every three to six months to avoid bacteria buildup, which can lead to eye infections.

* the basic eye

1 fill in brows

2 light shadow all over lid, from lashline to brow bone

3 medium shadow on lid, from lashline to crease

4 deeper medium shadow in crease, blending slightly above and below crease

5 liner all around eyes, meeting at the outer corner

6 black mascara top and bottom

1 fill in brows

4 deeper medium shadow

3 medium shadow

2 light shadow all over

5 liner all around

6 black mascara

TECHNIQUES FOR THE EYES YOU HAVE: SHAPES

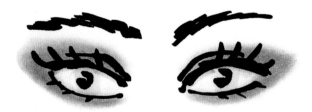

CLOSE TOGETHER

Try creating a winged effect with both shadow and liner. Extend a light shadow color up and out beyond the eye. Apply an extra dab of the light shadow on the inner lower lids to give the illusion of distance between the eyes. A deeper eye shadow layered in the crease and out to the wing will open up the eyes. This illustration shows gray shadow as the base color with navy blended on top for depth.

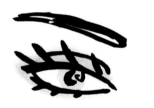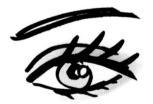

FAR APART

Anything goes, except for winged shadow or winged liner, which will make your eyes look wider. If you line your eyes, make the line thick on the top. If you line the bottom as well, have the top and bottom lines meet at the outer and inner corner of the eyes so they appear closer together.

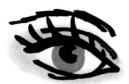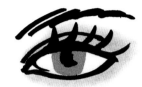

DEEP SET

Avoid dark shadow on the eyelid and in the crease as it will create too much depth. Light and sparkly shadows will work to highlight the lids. Apply one cool color all over the lid, from the lashline to just above the crease. Try placing the same shadow just below the eyes to really bring them out. Black liner and mascara are all you need to frame the eyes.

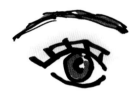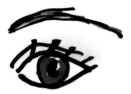

SMALL

Use a light eye shadow that is one to two shades lighter than your natural lid and apply all over your lid, from lash line to brow bone, with an eye shadow brush. Next, choose a medium shade that is one to two shades darker to blend into your crease. Add definition with tight, thin liner applied close to the lashes. Curling lashes and several coats of lengthening mascara will open up the eye.

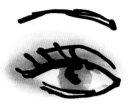
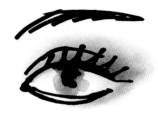

ALMOND-SHAPED

Liner will emphasize the beautiful shape of your eyes. To give the eye a lift, make the liner thickest on the outer corner. Lightly lining the bottom lash line will enhance your eye shape even more. For shadow, try a medium shade all over the lids from lash line to brow bone, with a darker color blended into the crease.

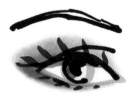
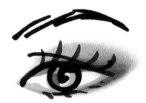

ASIAN

Create dimension with a light shadow like ivory or white all over the lid, from lash line to brow bone, and a medium tone in the crease and just above. Go for a fairly thick line with your eyeliner from the outer corner to the inner corner—you should be able to see it when you open your eye. Curling your lashes is a must.

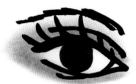 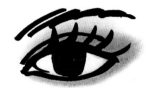

DARK BROWN

So many colors look gorgeous with brown eyes, including black plum, navy, and taupe. A strong, smokey eye with brown shadows is always gorgeous. The trick with dark brown eyes is to use a liner that is darker than your eye color, such as mahogany or espresso, to really make your eyes stand out.

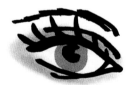 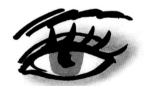

LIGHT BROWN

Light brown eyes are the most versatile and look gorgeous with a wide range of shadow colors. Choose medium browns in either warm or cool tones to bring out your eyes. For a foolproof look, go with brown or bronzey shadows. Black plum, navy, or dark brown liner will enhance the color of your eyes.

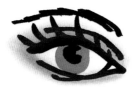
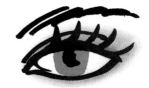

DARK BLUE

Brown shadows always work with deep-blue eyes, but slate grays and light purple shades will make your eyes look more exotic. Midnight blue and black liner will really define your eyes.

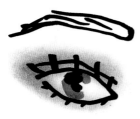
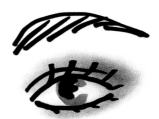

HAZEL

Hazel eyes are the chameleons of eye color. Bronzes, greens, or soft browns will all look beautiful. Warm browns or greens will make hazel eyes look green, while purple tones make them appear blue. A forest green all over the lid paired with a deep brownish black liner will bring out green tones and look amazing with your eyes.

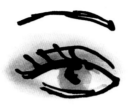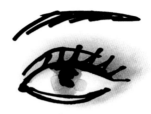

LIGHT BLUE/GRAY-BLUE

White, light gray, and lavender are the perfect cool tones to make blue and gray-blue eyes pop. Champagne or pale sparkles also look great. Navy and black liners will intensify the blue in your eyes even more.

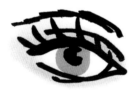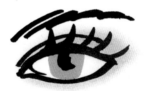

GREEN

Brown and plum shades such as taupe and heather perfectly complement green eyes. Avoid overly bright colors such as blue as they can take away from your eye color. Deep black-brown liner will make green eyes stand out even more.

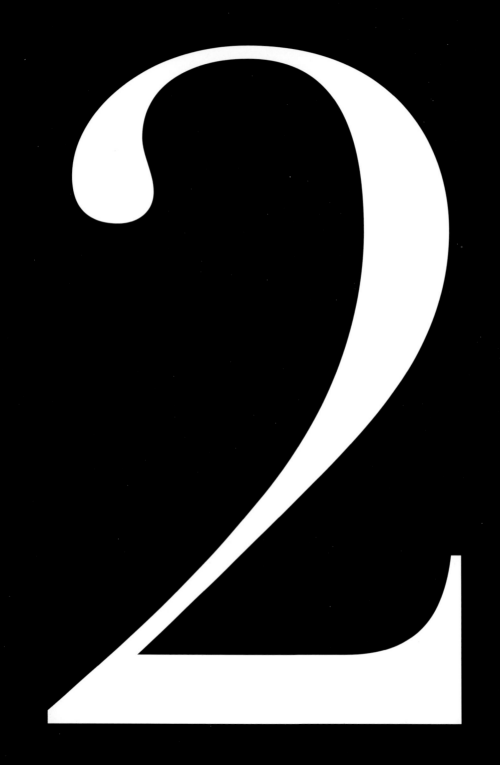

get
the
look

Changing your eye makeup transforms your whole look. A nude eye with a black gel liner is always sexy and gorgeous (and one of my favorite looks). Here are ten more go-to looks I love.

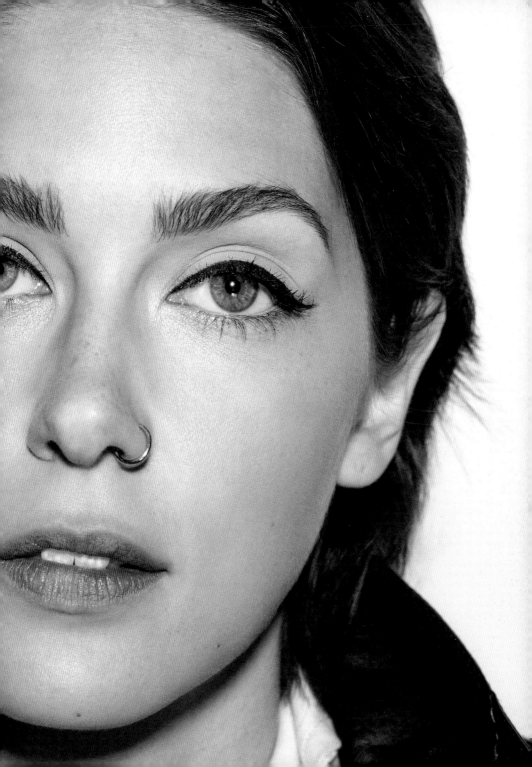

clean

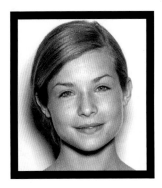

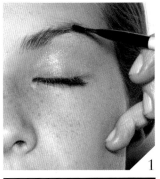

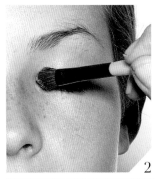

Sometimes all you need is a beautiful shimmer shadow and mascara and you're out the door. This look is gorgeous enough for daytime and elegant enough for a party.

Fill in the brows with an angled brow brush and powder. Keep your brows natural for this look.

Sweep shimmery beige or champagne shadow all across the lids from the lash line to just above the crease using an eye shadow brush.

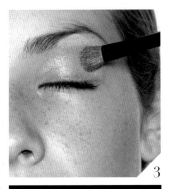

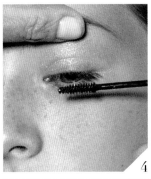

For added depth, apply a slightly darker shimmer shadow in the crease using a flat eye shadow brush.

Finish with two coats of black mascara.

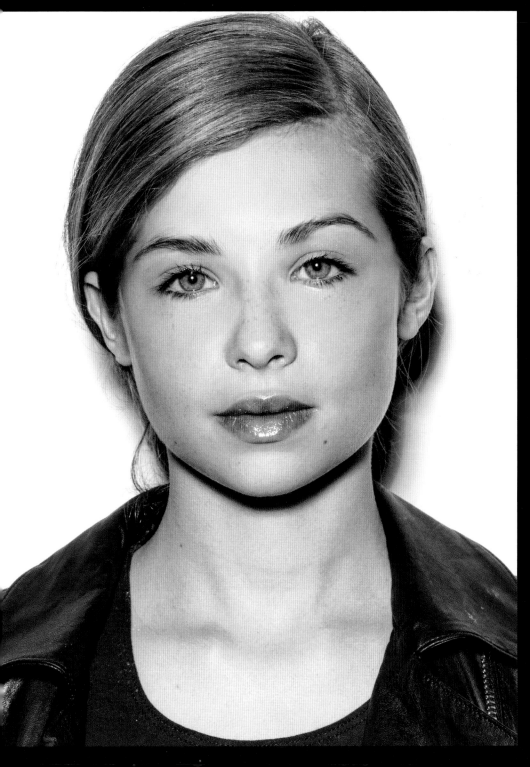

sparkly

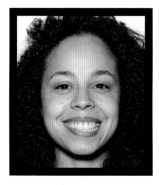

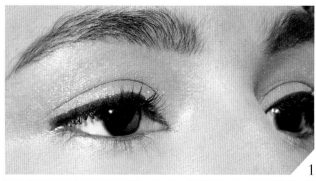

1

Pale hues open up and brighten your eyes. Add some shimmer for a pretty and festive look that works day or night.

With a cream shadow brush, layer an ivory-hued long-wear cream shadow all over the lid. This will provide a base coat that will last for hours.

From the lash line to just above the crease, apply a light-reflecting sparkle shadow all over the lid. We used a silvery-white shade.

To define eyes, apply a black long-wear gel liner with an ultra-fine eyeliner brush close to the lash line from the outer corner all the way across the top.

Finish with three coats of a volumizing mascara.

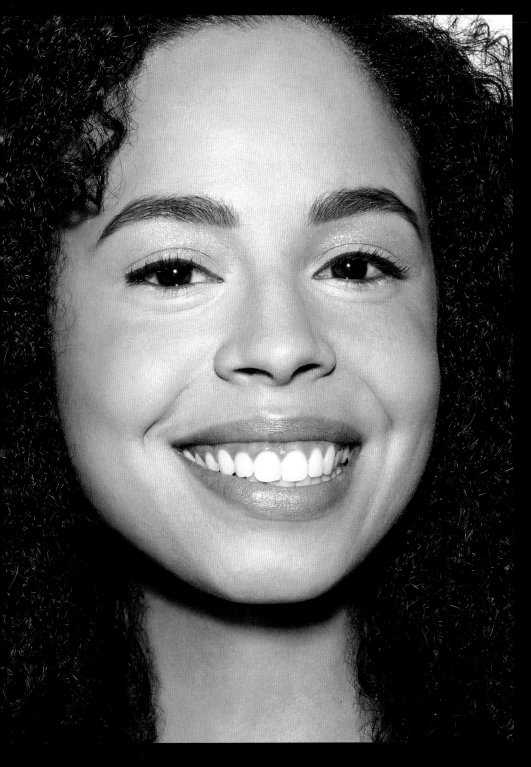

nude

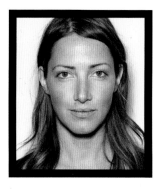

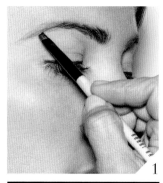

1

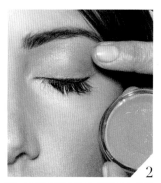

2

Using the same dusty rose shade on lips, cheeks, and eyes creates a gorgeous and glowy look. It's also incredibly easy to pull off.

With an angled brow brush, apply an eye shadow in the same tone as your hair color to the brows. Apply from the inner corner of your brows and brush straight up. Continue to brush up and over through the arch and on to the end with light strokes, filling in any gaps.

On Chelsa, we used a dark gray-brown.

Using your fingers, sweep pot rouge in a dusty rose shade over the lower lid to add a soft hint of color to the lids. For subtle shimmer, we layered a champagne shimmer shadow on top with an eye shadow brush.

Apply a deep black-brown long-wear eyeliner with an ultra-fine eyeliner brush. Place close to the lash line from the outer corner all the way across.

Finish with two coats of thickening mascara.

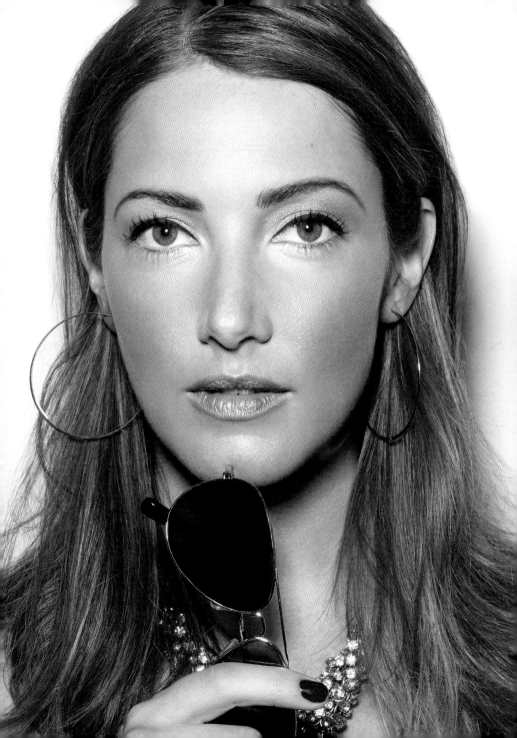

bronzed

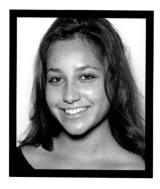

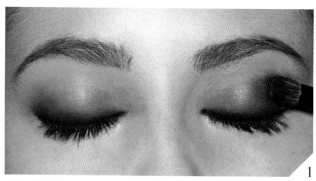

1

For a modern take on the sun-kissed look, apply warm bronzy hues on eyes, cheeks, and lips.

Using an eye shadow brush, apply bone shadow all over the lid, from lash line to brow bone. Apply a soft terra-cotta shadow on the lid, blending just above the crease. Layer shimmery bronzy brown shadows, placing the color close to the lash line with an eye shadow brush. Make sure to blend so there are no lines. You want the darker color to be closest to the lash line.

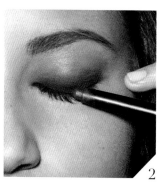

2

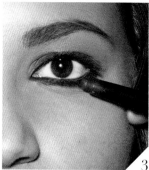

3

Use a rich brown cream shadow stick as your eyeliner and apply as close to the upper lash line as possible, practically rimming the eye. Start your liner from the outer corner and draw a soft line toward the inner corner.

Repeat on the lower lash line, moving from the outer corner all the way across. Blend and diffuse with a flat eyeliner brush to soften the lines even further. Finish with three coats of volumizing mascara.

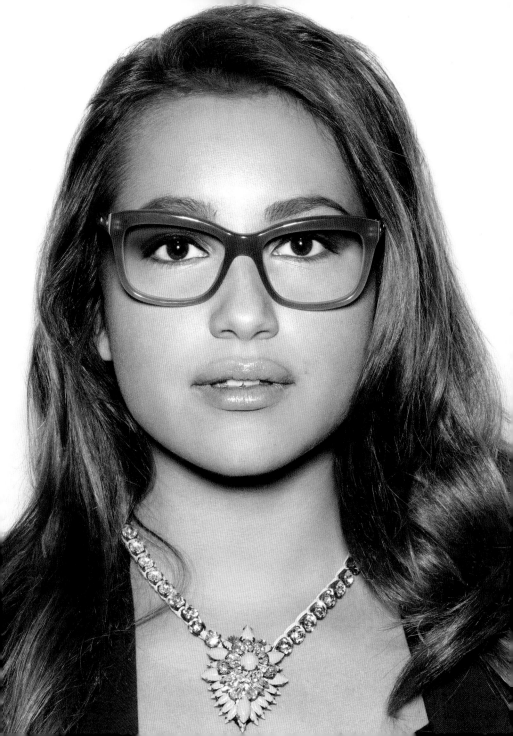

fun

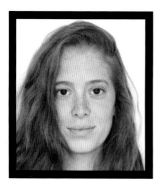

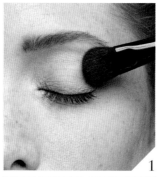

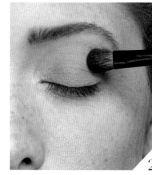

A foolproof way to use bold shadow: pair it with black liner and mascara, and keep the rest of the face neutral with soft blush and nude lips. I love how this lavender works with Ella's hair and eyes.

Apply a sheer white shadow all over the lid with an eye sweep brush as a base color. Place the shadow from the lash line to the brow bone.

With an eye shadow brush, apply a medium shade of a fun shadow color from the lash line to slightly above the crease. Apply the same shadow underneath the lower lashes with an eye smudge brush.

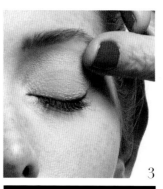

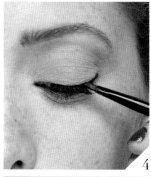

Layer a brighter shade of the same hue (in this case a brighter shade of lavender) on top of the colored shadow, from lash line to slightly above the crease, for additional depth. Using your fingers to apply will result in a denser application.

Apply a very thin line of black gel eyeliner with an ultra-fine eyeliner brush very close to the lash line from the outer corner all the way across. This will add definition. Apply three coats of black lengthening mascara to finish.

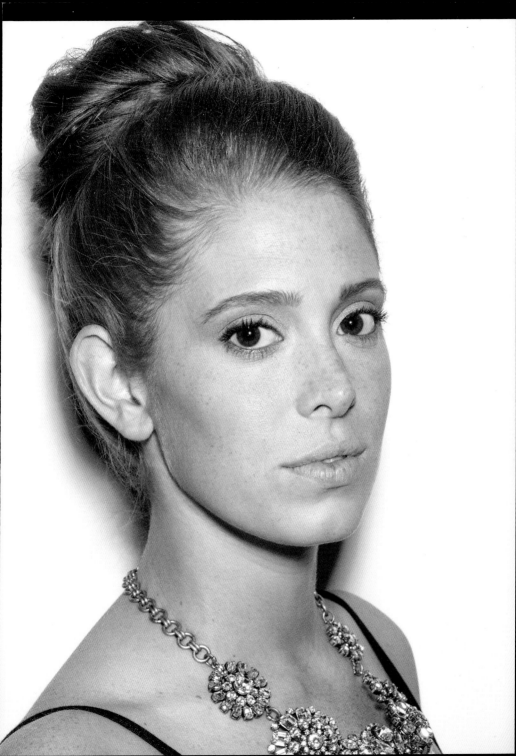

winged

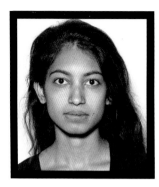

Dramatic and sexy, black winged liner always makes a statement and puts the spotlight on your gorgeous eyes.

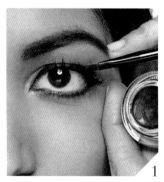

To make sure winged liner stands out, always apply after shadow. Apply black gel liner with an ultra-fine eyeliner brush from the outer corner all the way across the upper and lower lash lines.

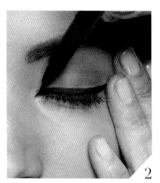

Turn black ink eyeliner on its side and, in smooth long strokes, draw a line from the inner corner across the upper lash line. The liner should get wider as you go across.

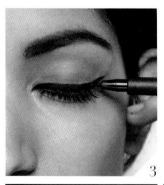

To create the wing, continue the line on the upper lid so it goes up and out past the outer corner of the eye. The end of the wing should taper to a soft point. You should be able to see the wing when you open your eyes—make sure the two sides match!

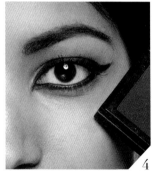

With an eye smudge brush, apply black powder shadow over your eyeliner on the lower lash line for a soft, smudged effect. Finish with three coats of black volumizing mascara.

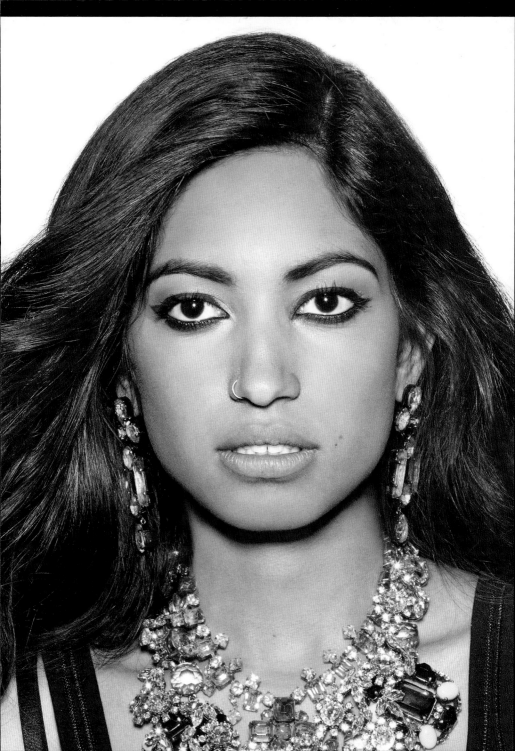

gilded winged

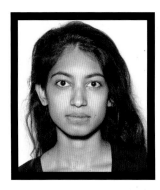

For a cool and playful take on winged liner, create a thicker, extra-long wing and add a sweep of vibrant gold shimmer.

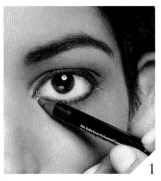

1

Use a black pencil liner to line around the eye, making sure the line is drawn all the way across both above and below the eye. Connect the lines at the inside corner of the eye.

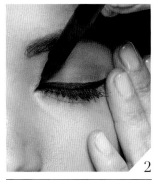

2

Use a black ink eyeliner as directed on page 64 to create the winged liner.

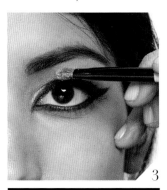

3

With an eyeshadow brush, apply a metallic gold eyeshadow on the lid just above the liner.

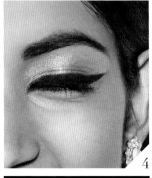

4

Continue applying the gold cream shadow from the top of the liner to just underneath the brow bone. Layer the pencil liner over the top line to keep it sharp. Finish with three coats of lengthening mascara.

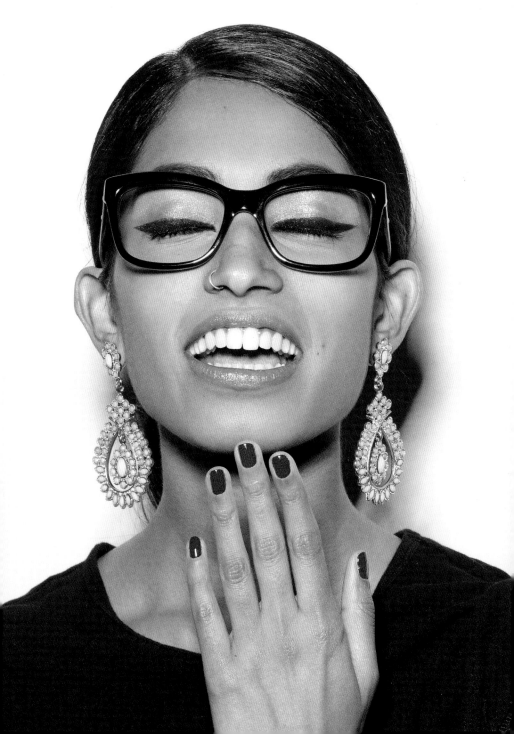

smokey

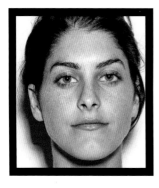

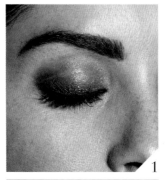

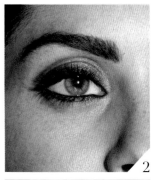

This is my sexy and cool take on the smokey eye.

Place a pale nude cream shadow all over the lid. Apply the base color from the lash line to just underneath the brow bone with a cream shadow brush.

Using the same brush, layer a silvery shimmer cream shadow all over the lower lid, building the density of the color from the lash line to the crease.

With an eye smudge brush, apply a shimmery slate color in the crease to add depth.

With a deep black long-wear eye pencil, line the entire upper and lower lash lines, making sure the lines meet in the outer corner. The lower line should be very thin and close to the lash line. Smudge the lines with a cream shadow brush.

Use an eyeliner brush to pick up color from the pencil, then use the brush to layer across the bottom lash line. Finish with three coats of black mascara.

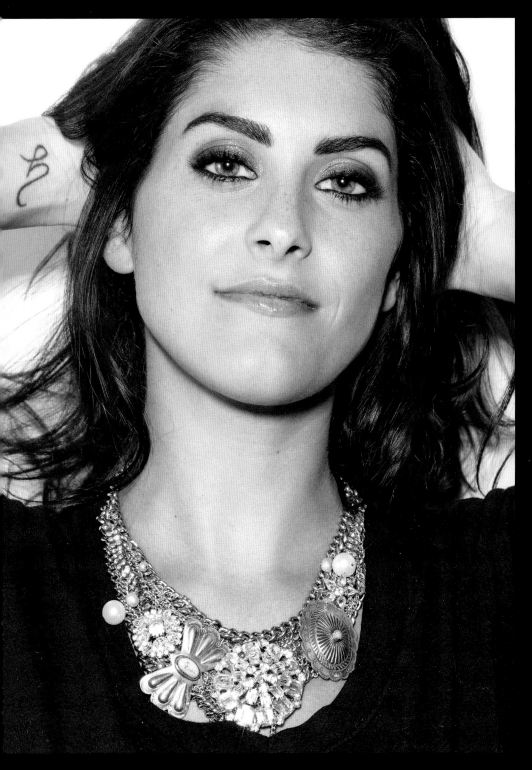

soft smokey

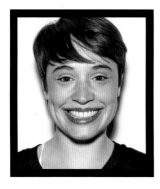

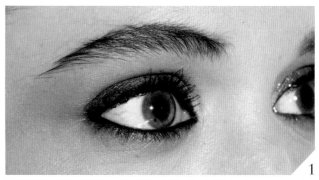

1

Smudged smokey warm hues make eyes pop.

Place a cream shadow in a pale nude color all over the lower lid with a cream shadow brush.

Using the same brush, layer bronze cream shadow all over the lower lid, building the density of the golden brown shimmer from the lash line to the crease.

With an ultra-fine eyeliner brush, apply a black gel eyeliner. Start from the outer corner and move all the way across the lid. Draw the liner just past the outer corner for a subtle winged effect.

With a flat liner brush, apply a black-brown shadow, layering it on top of the liner on the upper lid. Start from the outer corner and work your way all the way across. You want the line to be imperfect and slightly smudged. Then, with whatever is left on the brush, line the lower lash line. Finish with three coats of volumizing mascara to give the lashes thickness and volume.

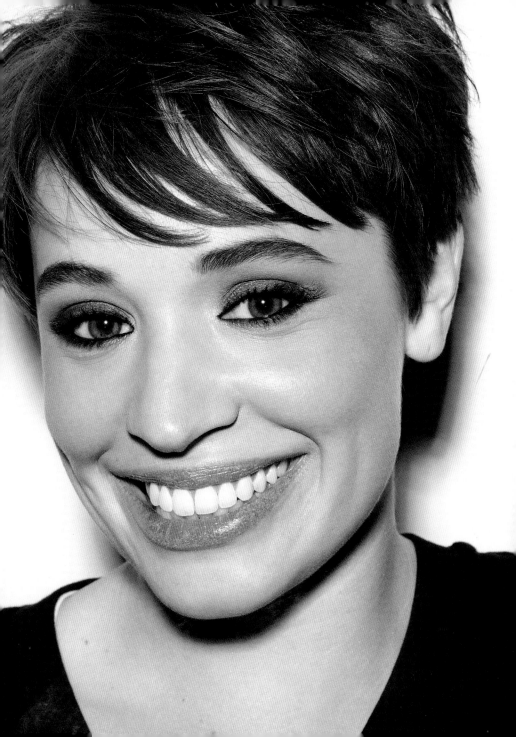

retro glam

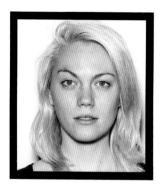

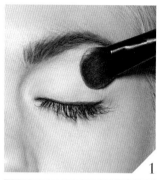

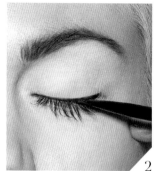

1

2

Hollywood starlet glamour is easier to achieve than you think. White shadow, gel liner, and a bit of red lipstick, and you're ready for your close-up.

Create polished and defined brows by applying eye shadow to the brows in a tone that complements your hair color. On Alissa we used soft gray-beige shadows that work with her ash-blonde hair. A clear brow gel completes the look, setting brows in place.

Apply white eye shadow all over the lid with an eye sweep brush. Layer the color from the lash line to the brow bone. With an eye shadow brush, layer even more on the lower lid to make the color more opaque.

To define eyes, use a deep inky blue gel eyeliner. Apply with an ultra-fine eyeliner brush very close to the lash line from the outer corner all the way across. A black liner would also work with this look, but I chose an inky blue shade to highlight Alissa's pretty blue eyes.

For ultra-dramatic lashes, apply false lashes (see page 74). Or apply three coats of black mascara. Before the lashes dry, gently press them up with your fingers to curl them.

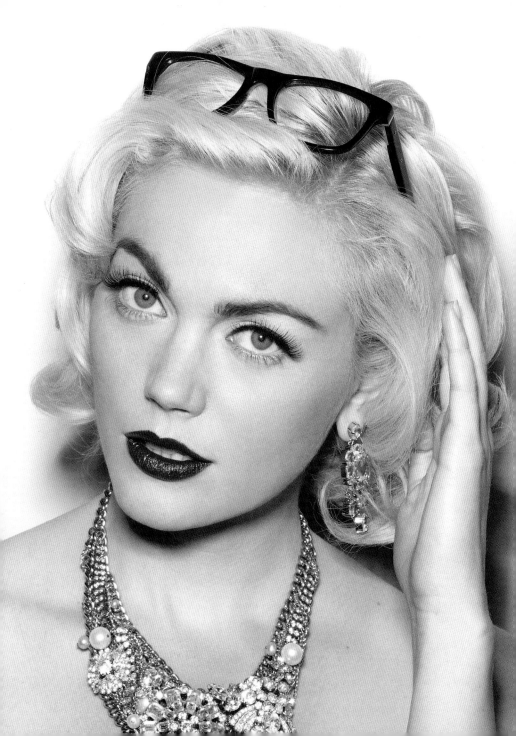

✱ false eyelashes

When you want to amp up your eyes and create a more glamorous or dramatic look, reach for the false eyelashes after you have done your makeup. You can find false lashes at any beauty supply store. It is helpful if your eyes are already lined prior to applying—the line acts as a marker for where to attach the edge of the lashes.

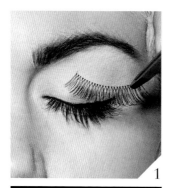

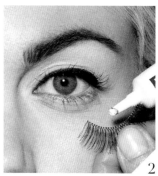

Compare the width of one of the false lashes with your own, holding it up to your lash line to see if they match. If it is too wide, you can snip a little bit off the outer corner with scissors to make it work. Repeat with the other lash.

Apply a thin line of lash glue straight from the tube to the entire base of the false lash.

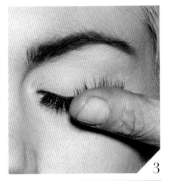

3

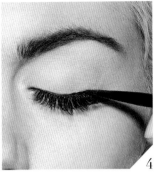

4

Use your fingers to place the false lash directly onto your eyelid at the lash line, adjusting it until it is in place. Hold it until it is dry.

Add an additional sweep of jet black gel or ink liner to the top lash line from the outer to inner corner.

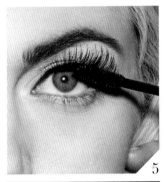

5

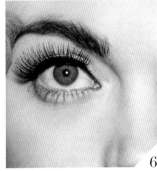

6

Once the glue is dry, add an extra coat of mascara to bind your real lashes to the false ones.

Repeat on the other side.

ONE GIRL, TWO LOOKS: GO BOLD ON LIPS OR EYES

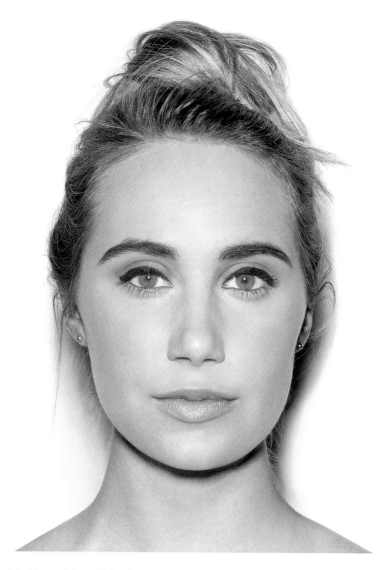

A bold eye with a soft lip always works. Here Gabriella rocks turquoise shadow, black gel liner, and black mascara paired with a nude lipstick and pale pink blush.

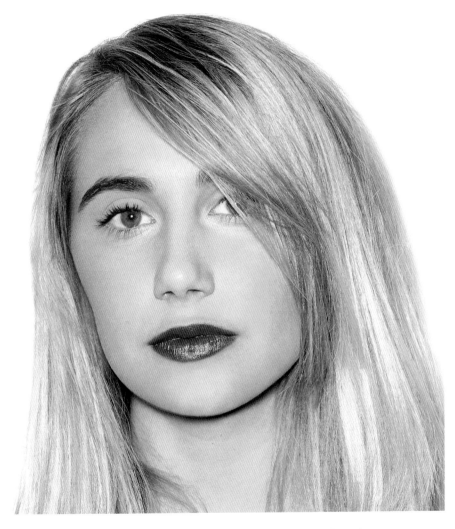

Bold lips with a clean eye looks totally fresh and modern. Go with a confident shade of red lipstick and just a sweep of mascara on lashes with a brighter blush.

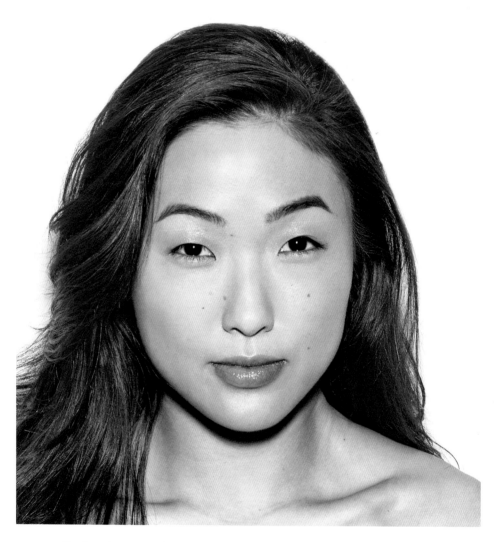

For day, choose a nude pink blush and a pinky beige lip color. On the eyes, apply ivory shadow on the lids paired with thin black gel liner on the upper lash line, thin pencil liner on the lower lash line, and black mascara.

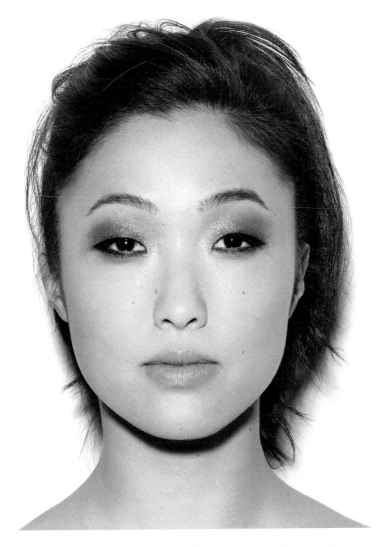

For night, just add a smokey eye. Sweep a dark gray-brown shadow from the lower lid to the crease. Layer a rich dark brown sparkle shadow from the lash line up to above the crease. To finish it off, smudge brown shadow just underneath the lower lash line.

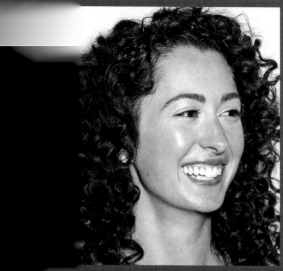

White shadow all over the lid is an easy trick to open up your eyes. Pair with lots of black mascara for a pretty look.

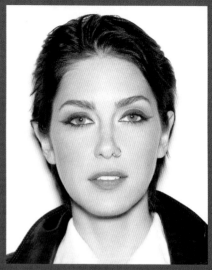

Ultra thick, winged liner in an intense cobalt blue adds instant edge.

Smokey brown shadow and black liner really bring out Alice's gorgeous eyes.

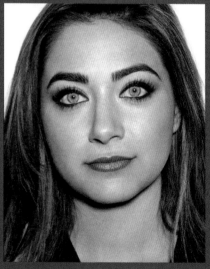

A mix of plum and brown shimmer shadows looks beautiful with Dana's bright blue eyes.

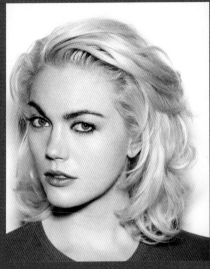

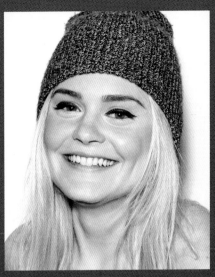

Sometimes liner all around the eye paired with black mascara has a very rock-star effect. Alissa pulls it off perfectly.

Isabelle's peaches-and-cream looks stand out with a thick brown liner.

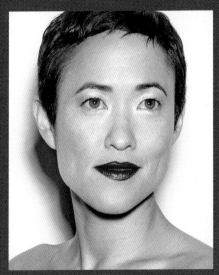

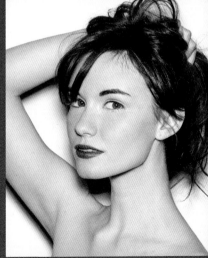

White shimmer shadow applied all over the lid and to the inner corners make M.C.'s eyes pop.

Angela's porcelain skin and rich brown hair look amazing paired with cranberry lips and a subtle lined eye.

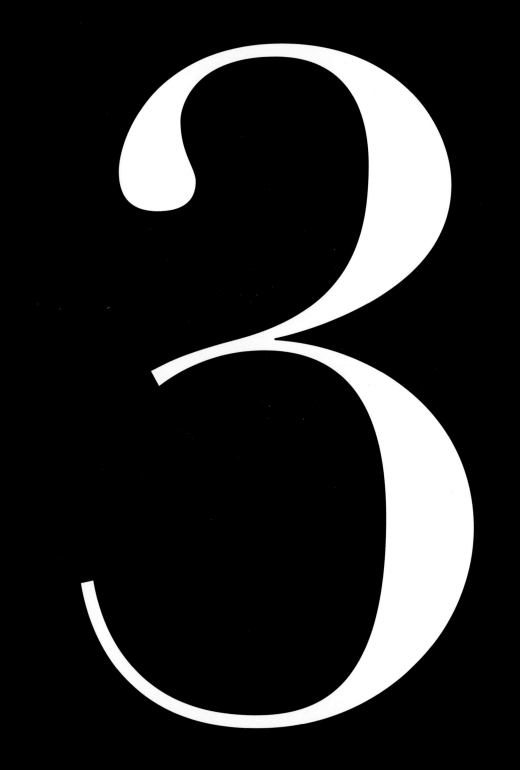

hey,
four-
eyes!

It's no secret that I love glasses. They offer an instant way to change up and enhance your look. Here's my take on finding the right pair and how to make your eyes stand out underneath your lenses.

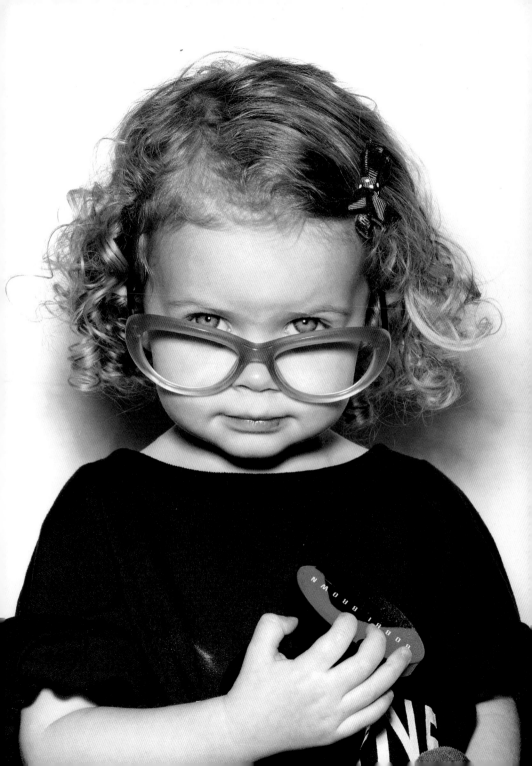

MY LIFE IN GLASSES

My own journey in glasses began in the '70s, when I sort of failed my eye test (the one with the bottom row of letters that is tough to read even if you have twenty-twenty vision). The doctor told me that I had the choice to get glasses or not. I immediately said yes to glasses. I had just seen Sissy Spacek host *Saturday Night Live* wearing the cutest round, wire specs, and I couldn't wait to get my own pair. Later, I switched to a pair of classic New England–prep tortoiseshell-rimmed glasses—perfect for my college days in Boston. I liked those glasses so much that I wore them in the photograph for our roomies' holiday card. When my mother received the card and saw the picture, she called laughing to ask if I was wearing those joke-shop nose-and-glasses. (Thanks, Mom.)

I wore glasses on and off for most of my early adult years—mostly when I was reading. Then right on cue, just before I hit forty, my eyesight changed and I needed glasses for distance and close-up. Not that it was necessarily bad news. Different lenses meant I got to play with different frames. After I had my third baby, I read an article about a new procedure called Lasik. The surgery took all of five minutes and I could be glasses-free (mostly). I chose to adjust my eyesight so that I could easily see my baby while he was in my arms. Once again, I'd only wear glasses for reading. That was until I saw Tina Fey, the epitome of the confident smart girl, rocking those black Superman frames. I headed straight to the store to get my own pair. The moment I tried on those black, heavy rims, I loved the vibe. I wanted to wear them all the time. I haven't taken my pair off yet.

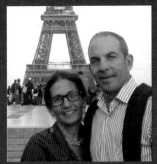 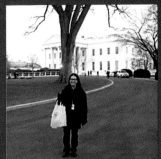 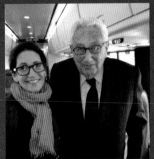

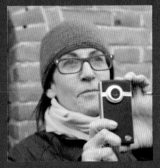 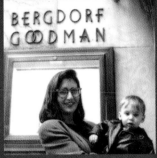 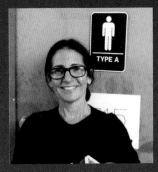

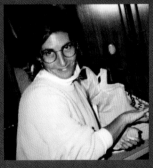 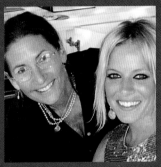 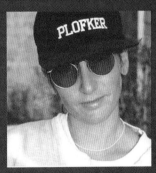

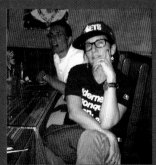 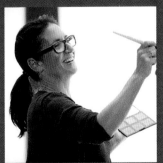 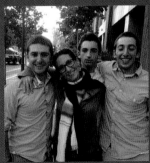

THE HISTORY OF EYEWEAR

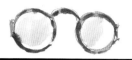
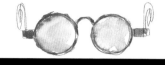
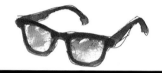

Spectacles—two framed round clear magnifiers bolted together with a rivet—arrive on the scene in Italy in 1289. Early frames are made of wood, iron, brass, leather, animal horn, bone, or tortoiseshell.

In 1740, European spectacle makers add temples—side arms that hook on to your ears—turning spectacles into glasses.

Trendsetters in the 1780s love lorgnettes, spectacles held with one long, decorative handle. This becomes a popular look for the opera.

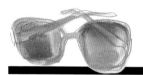
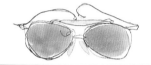
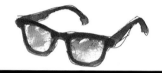

In 1929, Sam Foster of Foster Grant sells sunglasses on the boardwalk in Atlantic City. Once Hollywood starlets like Greta Garbo start wearing them a few years later, they become the hot accessory.

World War II aviator glasses are invented in 1941 to help fight the glare of the sun while flying at high altitudes.

Thanks to the rise of plastic frames in the 1950s, glasses become cheaper, allowing people to own several different pairs. Plastic square-rimmed glasses become popular for men, thanks to James Dean, Clark Kent, and Buddy Holly.

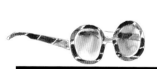
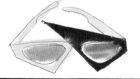
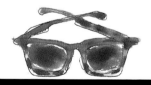

In the late 1960s and early 1970s, the fashion world recognizes the huge market potential for glasses, and brands such as Christian Dior and Pucci launch their own lines.

Fun and offbeat style rules the 1980s, with punk, asymmetrical, neon, and mismatched frames becoming popular.

Thanks to Tom Cruise and *Risky Business*, Ray-Ban Wayfarer sunglasses are everywhere in the early '80s. Three hundred sixty thousand pairs are sold in 1983 alone!

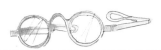 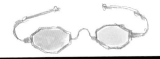

The oval or round metal frames popular in the 1700s become fancier as a status symbol: In Europe, the wealthy wear ivory, gold, or jewel-encrusted frames; in China, tortoise is favored for luck and longevity.

Colored lenses in smoke-gray, green, blue, and pink are trendy in Europe and China in the early 1800s.

In the mid-1800s, monocles are popular with politicians, professors, and anyone hoping to look intellectual.

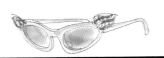 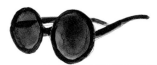 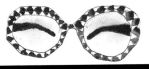

For women in the 1950s, Marilyn Monroe and other stars inspire the cat-eye glasses trend in both sunglasses and regular frames.

In the 1960s, Jackie O's big black round sunglasses become her trademark, starting a trend.

Graphic black-and-white frames inspired by 1960s Pop Art blur the line between glasses and art.

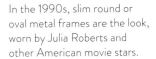 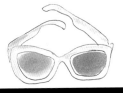 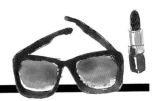

In the 1990s, slim round or oval metal frames are the look, worn by Julia Roberts and other American movie stars.

Downtown geek chic is epitomized with hipster glasses in the mid-2000s. Oversize pairs with thick plastic frames are seen on men and women alike.

In 2014, Bobbi Brown is the first makeup artist to launch her own eyewear line.

your perfect glasses

Glasses make an instant statement. To change up your look, you only have to change your frames. I've seen women look that much hipper, younger, and more confident just by putting on a new pair.

✳ how to choose glasses

STYLE Do you want trendy, hipster, chic, or classic? Go for whatever style you want; this is totally up to you.

FACE SHAPE Follow the guidelines for your face shape—oval, heart, round, or square—to find frames that will flatter your features.

FRAME THICKNESS Would you prefer glasses that make a statement (thick) or are more understated (thinner)?

COLOR Decide if you want frames that will brighten your face or enhance your skin tone. Do you want to go with neutral tones, nude shades, or would you prefer to add a pop of color? Always go with a hue you love.

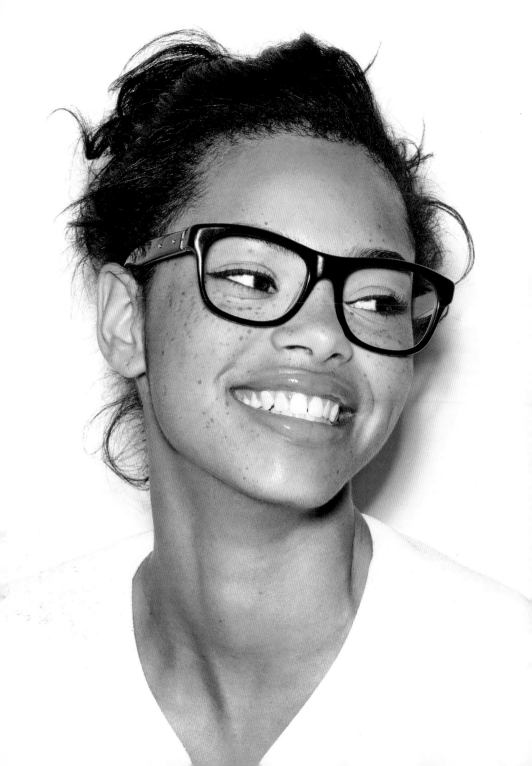

The secret to finding perfect glasses is to buy the ones you love. Glasses can be pricey, so take your time and try on a bunch of styles. If you're not sure which pair is for you, get another opinion. My son posted his frame choices on Facebook and his "friends" voted—a cool way to do it.

Finding the right glasses is not unlike choosing the best haircut for your face. First decide what style you like: simple, quirky, cool—there are endless options. Tear pictures from magazines or collect images on Pinterest. It helps to find frames you love on a face with a shape and coloring similar to yours. If you're not sure of your face shape, take a look in the mirror with your hair pulled back. Is your face oval, heart-shaped, round, or square? Then check out my guidelines for finding frames that flatter your face.

After finding the right style and shape, think about color. It is a little like playing with makeup. When you add color to your face, it enhances your look. Black and tortoiseshell traditionally look good on everyone, but don't stop there. Bold color can brighten up your skin. Hues that are complementary to your eye color will bring out your eyes. And I love nude, either on the inside of a classic black frame, as a surprise, or on the whole frame. Nude is both modern and classic and works on nearly everyone.

With so many great choices out there, here are some general tips and guidelines to simplify the process.

TIPS FOR CHOOSING GLASSES

- Eyes should be centered in each lens.

- Choose styles that are in proportion to your facial features. If you have a small nose, for example, don't overpower it with thick, oversize frames.

- Frame shapes that contrast with your face shape are most flattering. You don't want your glasses to be the same shape as your face.

- The top of your frames should follow the line of your brows. Avoid having your eyebrows be too much above, or below, the frames.

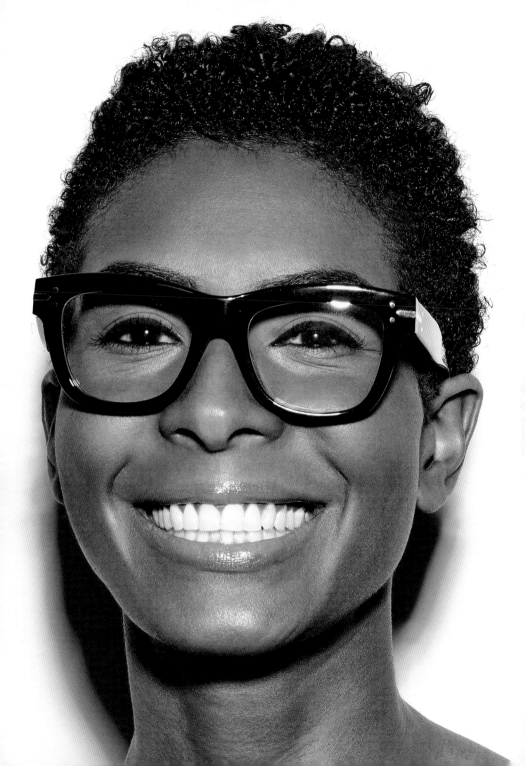

IF YOU HAVE AN OVAL FACE

You have a long and thin face with a chin slightly narrower than your forehead. Think Jennifer Aniston, Eva Mendes, Jada Pinkett Smith, and me.

GO FOR

- Glasses that are the same width as your face, not wider.

- Proportion! This is more important than frame shape for oval faces. Focus on frames that reflect the size of your features and face shape as a whole. So if you have small features, avoid thick, large frames. If you have larger features, avoid rimless frames that will get lost. It is all about balance.

- Variety! Most styles work well with your face shape, so have fun and mix it up.

AVOID

Narrow frames that will make your face appear longer, or way oversize frames that overpower your face.

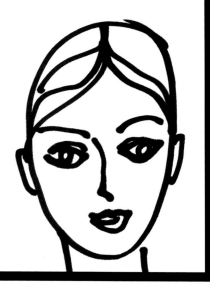

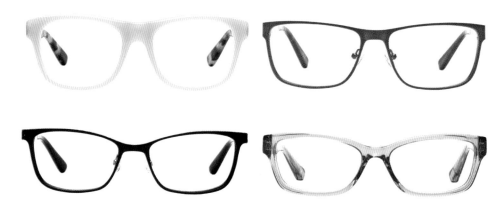

IF YOU HAVE A HEART-SHAPED FACE

You have an oval face that narrows at the chin, just like Jennifer Love Hewitt and Reese Witherspoon.

GO FOR

- Frames that are stronger on the bottom, to add the appearance of width to the lower, narrower part of your face.

- Oval frames that really emphasize your eyes.

- Both thick and thin frames work as long as they are in proportion with your features.

AVOID

Glasses that are weightier on top and put too much attention on the top of your face.

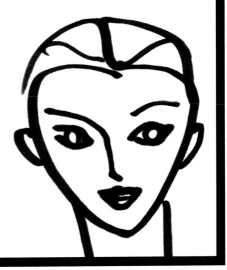

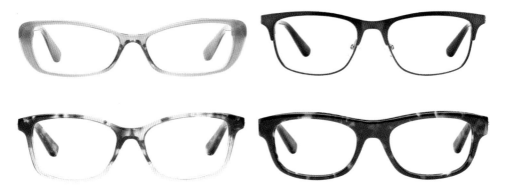

IF YOU HAVE A ROUND FACE

You have a fuller face, with a similar width and length. Think Mila Kunis and Cameron Diaz.

GO FOR

- Options with more angular lines. Square and rectangular frames are great choices.

- Cat-eye frames with upswept top corners will add a visual lift to your face.

- Temples that connect at the top corner of your frames draw the eye upward and balance fullness.

AVOID

Circular frames, especially smaller ones.

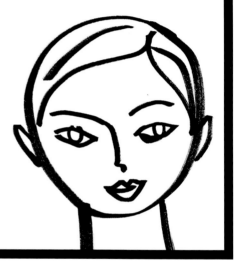

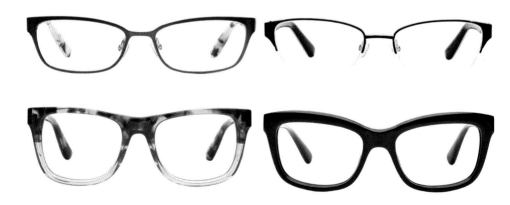

IF YOU HAVE A SQUARE FACE

You have a strong jawline and a broad forehead, just like Cate Blanchett, Sandra Bullock, and Oprah.

GO FOR

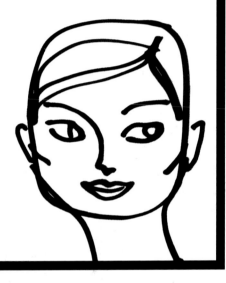

- Frames with curved or rounded corners to soften your strong face shape.

- Wide frames that extend out farther than the widest part of your face.

- Slimmer, lighter frames to soften your features.

- Round glasses. They look great because they contrast with your face shape. Just make sure they're in proportion to the size of your face: The larger your face, the larger the glasses should be if you're choosing round frames

AVOID

Thick dark frames with boxy, angular corners.

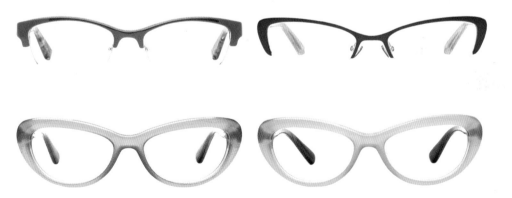

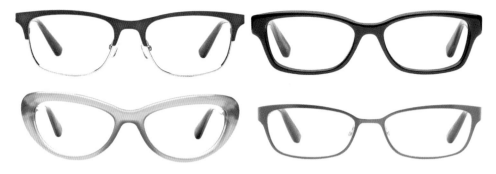

When you find a frame shape that works, get it in a variety of colors and styles.

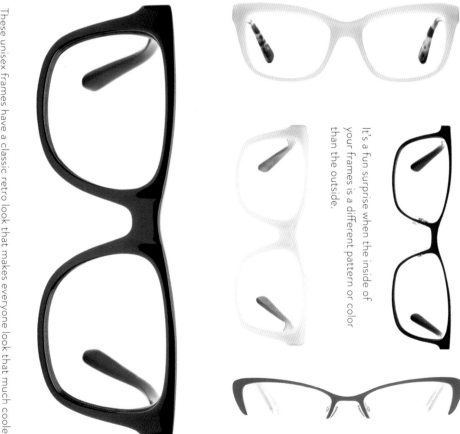

These unisex frames have a classic retro look that makes everyone look that much cooler.

It's a fun surprise when the inside of your frames is a different pattern or color than the outside.

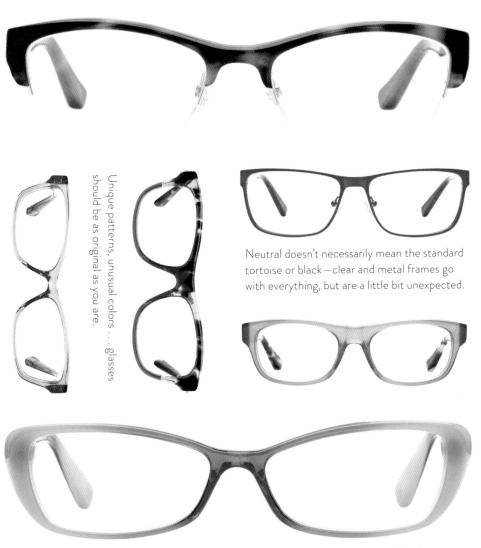

Unique patterns, unusual colors . . . glasses should be as original as you are.

Neutral doesn't necessarily mean the standard tortoise or black—clear and metal frames go with everything, but are a little bit unexpected.

Why choose just one color? This fun style has that funky ombre effect from caramel to dusty rose.

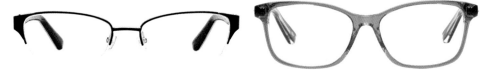

Think of glasses as an accessory—you should be armed with a few distinctive looks to suit your mood.

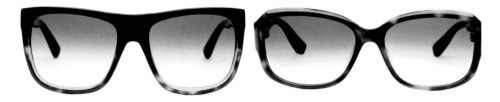

Tortoiseshell frames are universally flattering.

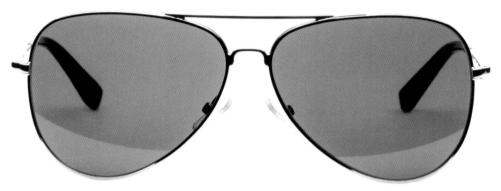

Aviators are that perfect combination of sporty and sexy.

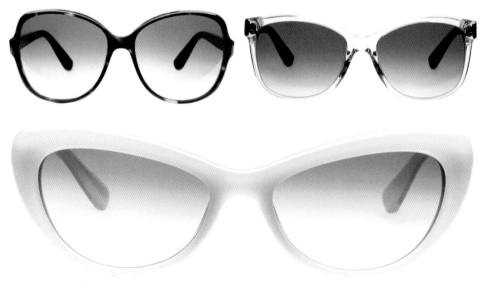

There is a playfulness to cat-eye frames that always lightens up your look.

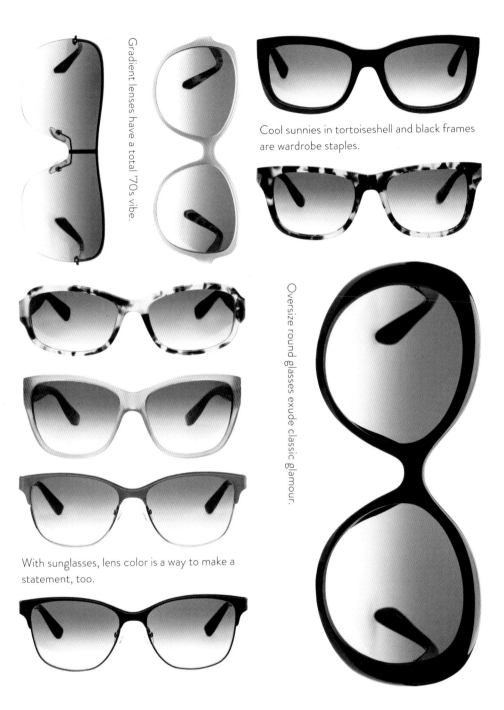

Gradient lenses have a total '70s vibe.

Cool sunnies in tortoiseshell and black frames are wardrobe staples.

Oversize round glasses exude classic glamour.

With sunglasses, lens color is a way to make a statement, too.

makeup for glasses

Glasses definitely make a style statement, but your eyes can get lost beneath your frames unless you adjust your makeup. Here are my favorite ways to make your eyes pop from behind your lenses.

* makeup tips for girls who rock glasses

- Eyeliner is key; it really adds definition from behind your lenses.

- Always define your brows with a shadow the same shade as your hair color. This will ensure that your glasses don't overpower your face.

- The glass in your frames can highlight undereye discoloration and darkness, so corrector and concealer underneath the eye and in creases is essential.

- Waterproof mascara won't smudge on your lenses.

- If you have strong frames, you can get away with stronger makeup.

- If your frames are delicate, or in a nude shade, don't let your makeup overpower your frames. Choose softer colors for shadow and create definition with a dark liner and mascara.

- The color of your eye shadow shouldn't compete with the color of your glasses. If you want to do the same color as your frames on your eyelids, try a base hue that's a shade lighter, and go a few shades darker for the crease color. Finish with black liner and mascara.

- For an easy look, go with a bold color on your lips and just corrector, concealer, and mascara for your eyes. Put on your glasses and you're done.

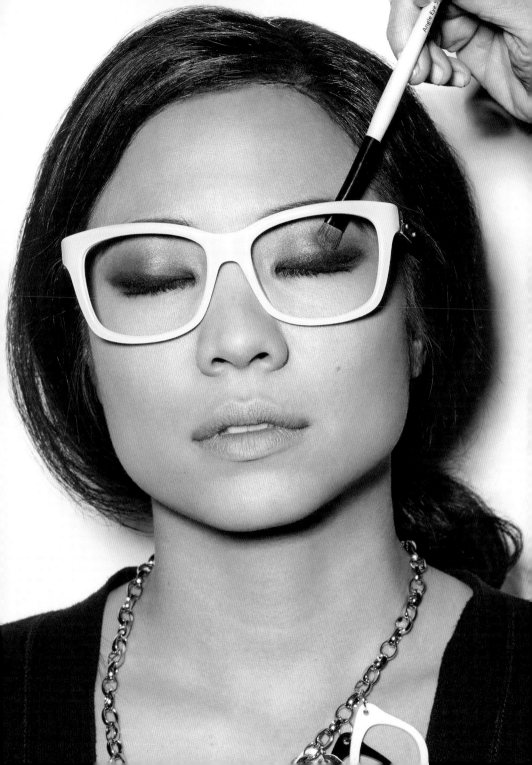

* basic makeup for glasses

* eye shadow that matches your hair color to fill in brows

* light base color shadow on the entire lid, from lash line to brow bone + a medium color on the lower lid, from lash line to crease

* gel liner on the top lash line

* thin line of powder liner to the lower lash line

* two coats of waterproof mascara

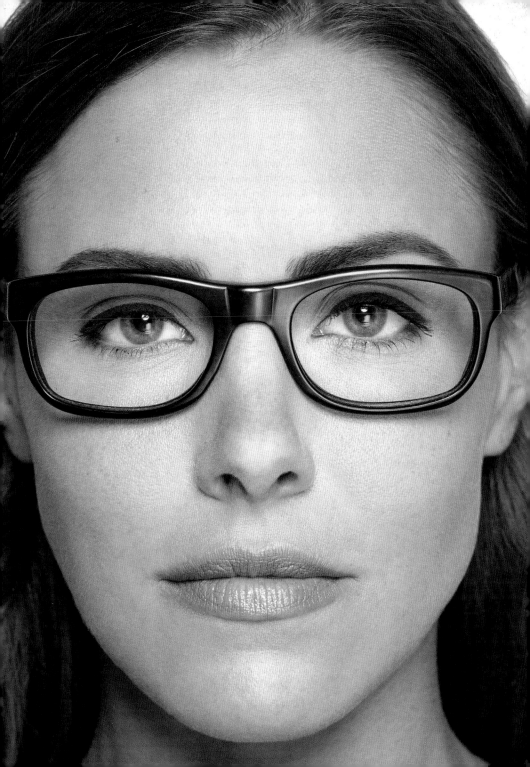

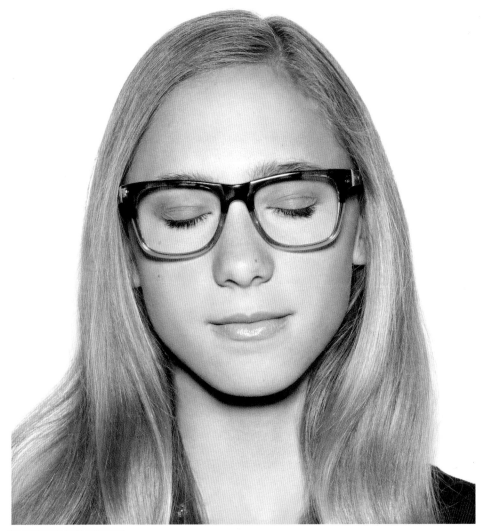

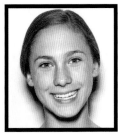

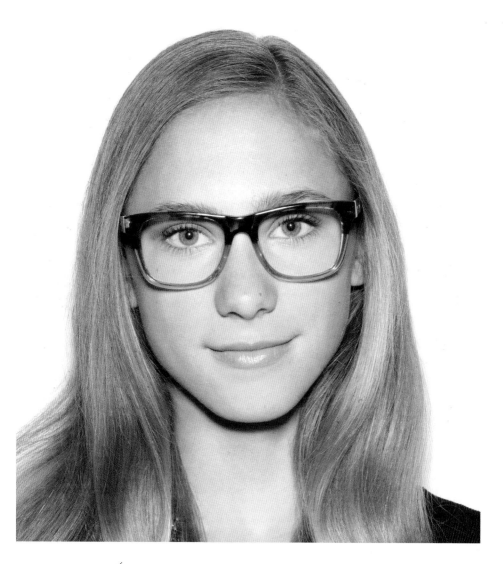

CRISTINA RENEE

An eye shadow color that is lighter and brighter than your frames will stand out, instead of competing with your glasses. A fun lavender shadow complements Cristina Renee's blue eyes and contrasts beautifully with her frames.

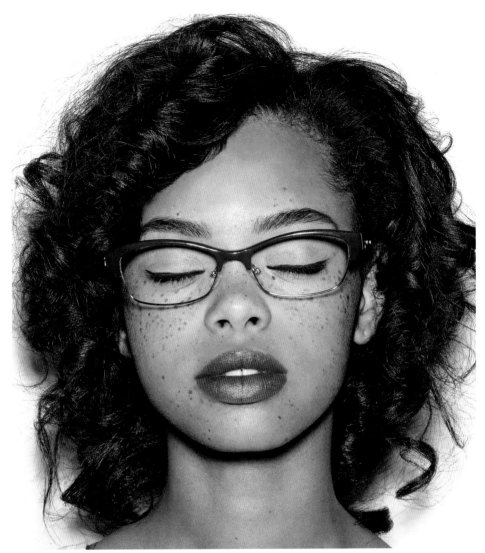

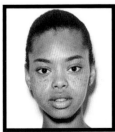

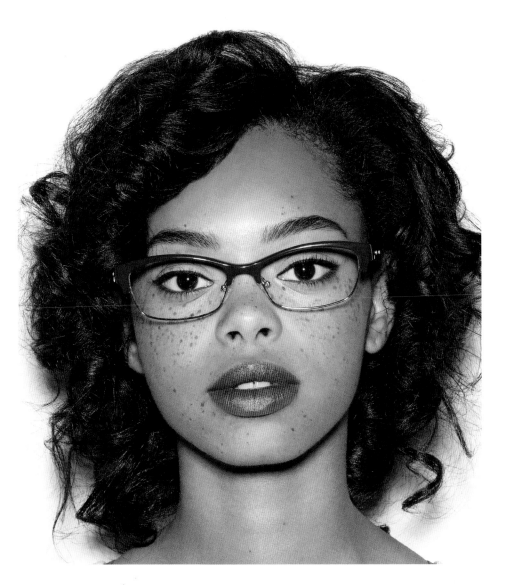

SABORNÉE

When you have a mix of confident colors on your hair, lips, and frames, keep your eye makeup simple and clean with only a little liner and mascara. Sabornée rocks burgundy hair, a super-bright pink lip, and thin navy top frames, so eye shadow isn't necessary.

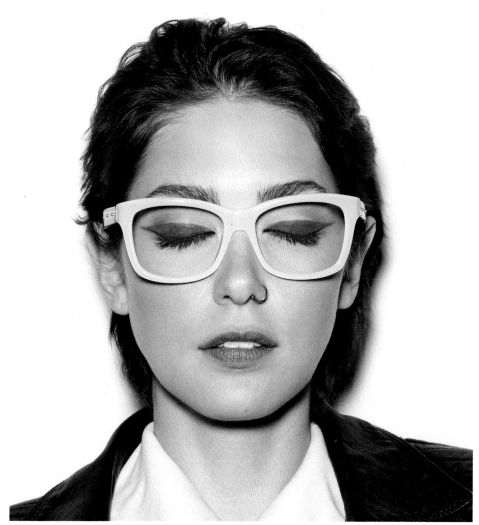

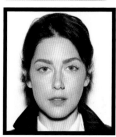

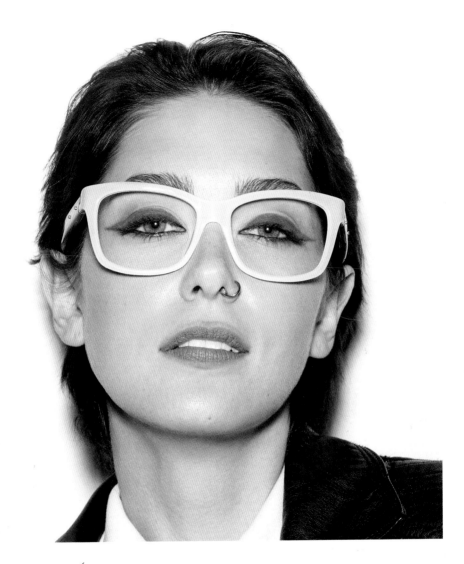

DANIELLE

White frames highlight both your eye and makeup colors, making them a great choice to pair with statement eye makeup. On Danielle, I did a modern take on screen siren Sophia Loren's iconic winged eyes, replacing the black liner with cobalt blue. Navy waterproof mascara completes the look.

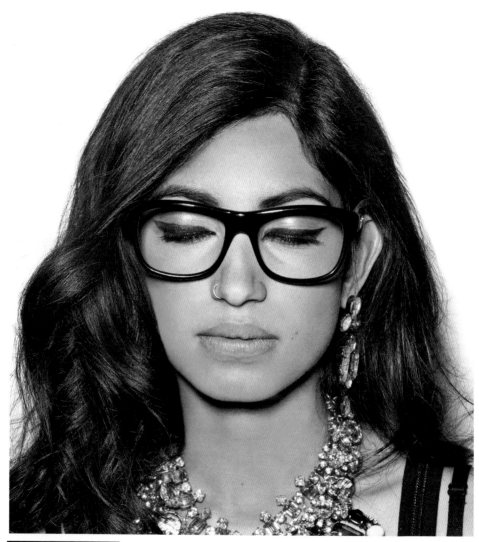

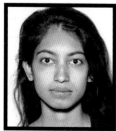

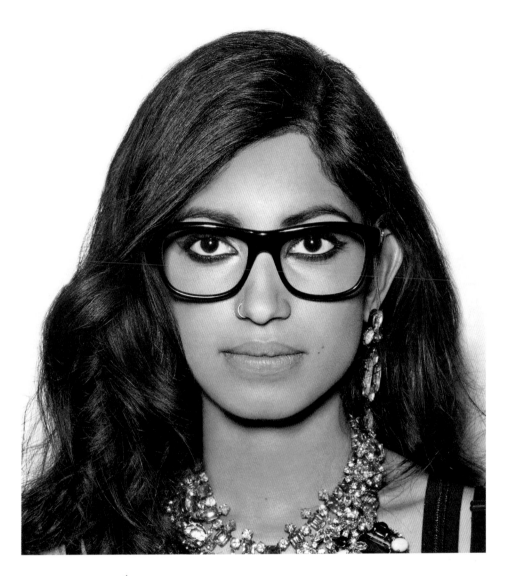

SARMISHTA

Bold liner, with minimal shadow, looks amazing with thick, oversize frames. Sarmishta wears strong, sexy winged liner in intense black, which makes her eyes pop beneath her glasses.

✳ choose your style

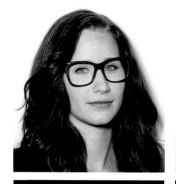 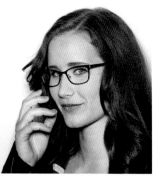

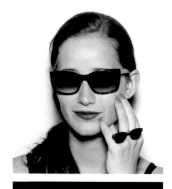 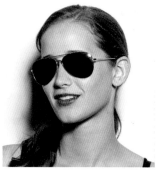

Use glasses to enhance your best features. On Emma, navy frames make her blue eyes stand out even more. Sleek, wide frames highlight her cheekbones. Tortoiseshell sunglasses look gorgeous with red hair. Aviator-style sunglasses paired with a red lip and a sleek ponytail show off a striking profile.

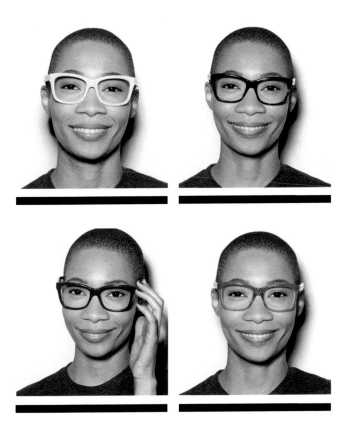

When you find a style that you love, get it in several colors.
These strong frames look amazing on Janicia in every hue. White
brightens her face, tortoiseshell is classic, navy pops beautifully,
while pink is soft and pretty, enhancing the natural color in
her cheeks.

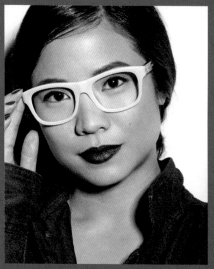

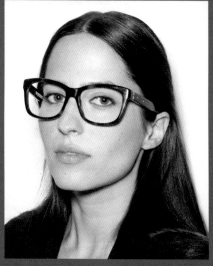

A bold red lip with a black jacket always works. To add a little more edge, throw on a pair of bold white glasses.

Oversize tortoiseshell frames with angular lines paired with subtle makeup and sleek hair looks polished, yet totally modern.

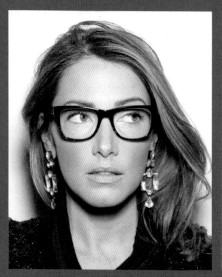

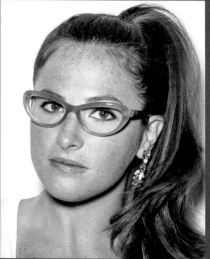

Preppy glasses look so cool with glamorous drop earrings and nude lips.

Sheer pink winged glasses are subtle yet stylish. They look great with a fun high ponytail.

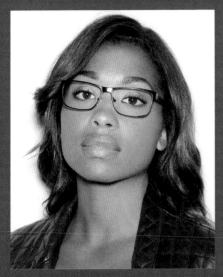

These wire tortoiseshell frames look great on Morgan—not overpowering yet still stylish.

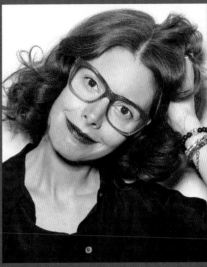

Refinery29 cofounder Christene Barberich has innate style. For a similar standout look, reach for bright frames and bold lips.

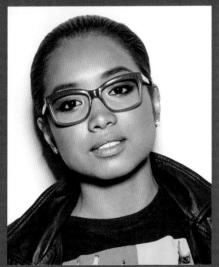

Tia's angular, wide frames flatter her face shape. The soft brown color looks perfect on her skin.

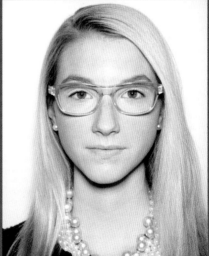

Lena's delicate coloring is enhanced with baby-pink sheer frames, pale pink lips, and pink pearls.

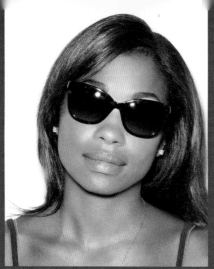

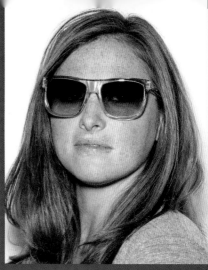

I love these upturned frames on Morgan. The tortoiseshell is chic and modern.

These bronzy pink oversize frames look adorable on Liz. Pink tones look great on a freckled face.

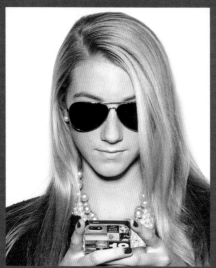

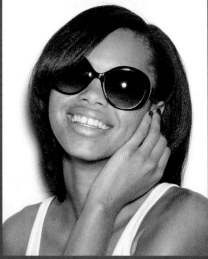

Lena is rocking the iconic aviators. I've yet to meet someone who doesn't look great in them.

"Pop star" is what I think when I look at Sabornée. These stylish frames are very now.

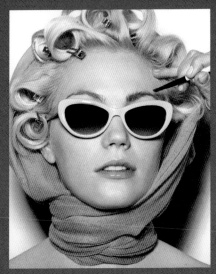

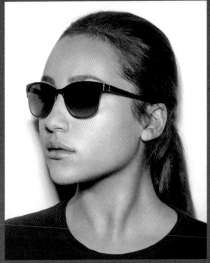

Retro sunglasses are cool and look fabulous on Alissa's face. The nude pink color is very flattering.

Nadia looks very chic in these shades. Simple and not overpowering, they work with every face shape.

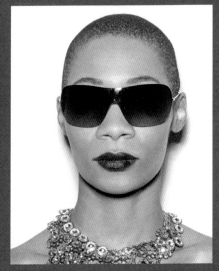

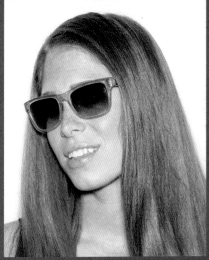

Rimless wrap frames exude an edgy and sophisticated vibe.

These pink frames are adorable with Ella's red hair and freckles.

thank you so much to everyone who worked on this amazing project.

BOBBI BROWN OFFICE
Alexis Rodriguez
Brielle Oliastro
Corinne Zadigan
Donald Robertson
Dorothy Mancuso
Elisa Munda
Jacob Simonson
Katie Brennan
Kelly Grgich
Lily Saltzberg
Mallory McLoughlin
Marie Claire Katigbak
Maureen Case
Nadia Morehand
Natalie Haimo
Sacha Gross
Tara Tersigni
Veronika Ullmer

MAKEUP ARTISTS
Cassandra Garcia
Danielle Lopes
Dillon Peña
Eduardo Ferreira
Eliano Bon Assi
Kim Soane
Lindsey Jackson
Marc Reagan
Rogelio Reyna
Tanya Cropsey
Tia Hebron

MODELS
Alice Anoff
Alissa Bourne
Althea "Tia" Cadavillo
Alyssa Ciccotti
Ana Diaz
Angela Neal

Brandy Joy Smith
Caroline Earley
Chelsa Skees
Christene Barberich
Cristina Renee Pliego
Dana Salah
Danielle Leder
Diane Duong
Elizabeth Sardinsky
Ella Crowe
Emma Lenchner
Gabi Dolce-Bengtsson
Isabelle Alsop
Janicia Francis
Kimberly Sardinsky
Lena Jewett
Liz Sardinsky
Marie Claire Katigbak
Morgan Booker
Nadia Morehand
Narvie Rundlet
Sabornée Judge
Samantha Yu
Sarah Morrissey
Sarmishta Mahendra
Sophia Corriere
Susannah Schaffer
Tara Tersigni

CHRONICLE BOOKS TEAM
Christine Carswell
Doug Ogan
Laura Lee Mattingly
Liza Algar
Pamela Geismar
Sara Schneider
Yolanda Cazares

WRITING
Sara Bliss

PHOTOGRAPHERS
Ben Ritter
Brian Hagiwara (products)
Henry Leutwyler (cover)

PHOTOGRAPHY ASSISTANTS
Andrew White
Danielle Leder

HAIR
Ahbi Nishman
Alicia Acuna
Kimberly Lemise
Michael Dueñas

NAILS
Roza Israel

SAFILO TEAM
Jennifer Earley
Kelly Kahn
Robin Scheer Ettinger
Ross Brownlee
Tatiana De Arruda Penteadò

FOOD
Falafel Hut
Jane Yaguda

TRANSPORTATION
Crestwood Limousine
Ron Hill

STUDIO
18 Label Studios
David Genova
Elizabeth Sardinsky

ENTERTAINMENT
Biggie
Caroline Earley
Maggie
Pup Pup

3 1333 04203 5780